TABLE OF CON

CW01507567

THE ULTIMATE GUIDE TO MENOPAUSE

7 EASY STEPS TO ACHIEVE SYMPTOM RELIEF, WEIGHT LOSS, AND HOLISTIC WELLNESS TO CONFIDENTLY EMBARK ON YOUR STRESS-FREE JOURNEY

HERA BENNETT

"Menopause is a time to tap into our wisdom and power."

— *JENNIFER RITCHIE PAYETTE*

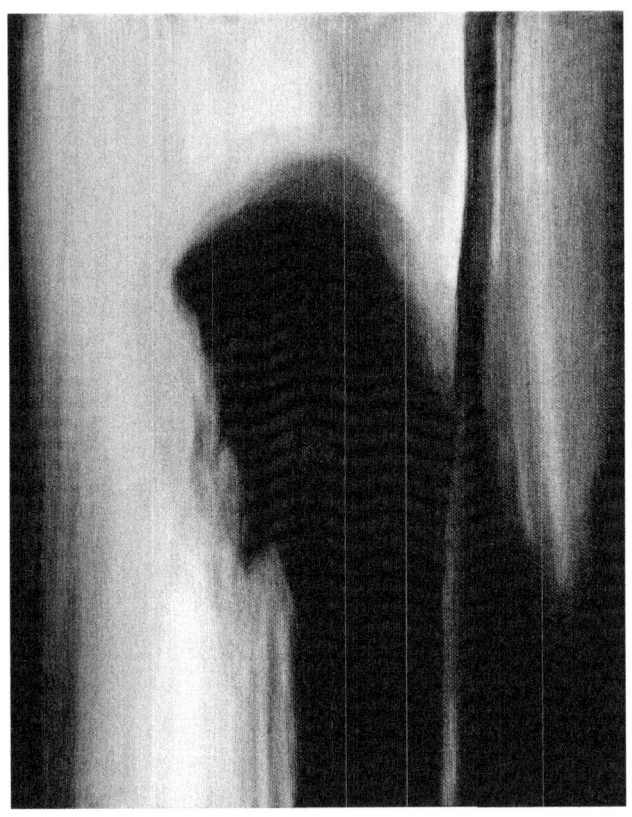

'Home', oil on canvas. © copyright Ngai Ning Yu 2023

INTRODUCTION

"Fireworks." That's what my friend Joey will tell you if you ask her how things are at the moment—and I believe her. Not long ago, I was there myself. Joey has an 11-year-old daughter, Lucy, who has just reached puberty, and she is everything but rainbows and sunshine. To make it worse, Joey has recently entered an early phase of menopause at age 46. Mood swings are flying around like firecrackers in their house, and Joey's husband and son are trying to avoid being hit.

In this whirlwind of hormones and unkind words flying left, right, and center, Joey is urgently seeking a way to manage menopause and support Lucy through puberty. She knows the feeling of being confused and alone when these life-altering changes happen. It's a journey all women go through, in many cases alone, and it's time to shed light on it so she can find the support she needs.

Picture this: You're lying in bed—struggling to sleep—and a sudden heat wave washes over you, leaving you drenched in sweat. Your heart is racing, and you're sure that you're dying. You're not alone. Women worldwide have this same experience—hot flashes, the unwelcome guests of the night. As you catch your breath, you glance in the mirror with worried eyes, fixating on the signs of aging and thinning hair.

That's exactly why I've written *The Ultimate Guide to Menopause*— to help women who are going through or will be going through what myself, Joey, and so many others have experienced. Together, we can navigate the intricate web of menopause and, yes, even find the calm and patience to deal with other life challenges, such as supporting adolescents and managing other relationships, one step at a time.

Menopause brings unspoken challenges, but the real problem here is that a lack of information and education adds to our confusion and anxiety. Think about it: As a teenager, you were prepared for puberty in one way or another, but no one sits you down to "pause" and prepare you for the big M—menopause!

Hot flashes, mood swings, and sleep troubles will disrupt your life. These effects aren't just physical; they can also cast an emotional shadow over you. Finding reliable methods for relief means adjusting your lifestyle, considering medication, or exploring tailored therapies.

Emotional ups and downs, anxiety, and depression affect us too. Mental support and coping strategies are vital, from counseling to self-help techniques.

Self-esteem and self-confidence can waver as our bodies and emotions change. Support networks and counseling can guide our journey of self-discovery.

Relationships face many challenges during menopause. How do you adapt to keep relationships healthy throughout this phase in your life?

You aren't alone. Your challenges are shared by countless women. True to the warrior that you are, it's time to seek understanding and find support.

I'm a woman in my early 50s, a mother of two wonderful girls, and an experienced breastfeeding mother who has dedicated herself to supporting other moms in their breastfeeding journeys. Now, as my children are stepping into early adulthood, I find myself drawn to helping other women navigate their own menopause experiences.

My journey, like many of yours, wasn't always smooth when this phase hit. I wasn't fully prepared, and the confusion and discomfort were very real. This experience has fueled my passion to break down the stigma surrounding menopause and reshape the narrative around this natural phase of life. Writing this book wasn't just a career choice for me; it's a heartfelt calling, and I'm excited to inspire and uplift women worldwide.

In *The Ultimate Guide to Menopause*, I will provide you with practical advice, evidence-based information, and emotional support to make sure you never feel alone during this phase of your life. You'll uncover a wealth of information on the following topics:

- **Understanding your changing body:** You'll better understand the intricate changes happening to your body, empowering you with the knowledge you need to navigate this natural transition with awareness and confidence.
- **Finding relief and coping:** Delve deep into the numerous symptoms of menopause and explore effective coping strategies, which range from natural remedies to hormonal therapies.
- **Learning the power of physical activity:** Discover the transformative effects of exercise in alleviating

menopausal challenges. Learn about a variety of workouts designed to invigorate both your body and soul, helping you maintain vitality and overall well-being.

- **Exploring nutrition and weight management:** Understand the pivotal role of nutrition in managing the menopausal transition. Get expert guidance on tailoring your diet to address hormonal imbalances and achieve your weight loss goals.
- **Nurturing relationships and intimacy:** Discover strategies for nurturing intimacy and deepening connections with your partner during this transformative phase. Find out how to reignite the flames of passion and maintain fulfilling relationships.
- **Empowering yourself and others:** Learn how to harness your newfound knowledge to become a beacon of empowerment, not just for yourself but also for others navigating the challenges of menopause.
- **Fostering inner harmony and resilience:** Explore the emotional and spiritual aspects of menopause and gain insight into ancient wisdom and mindfulness practices that can help you cultivate inner harmony and resilience, guiding you through the emotional ups and downs.
- **Embracing menopause with confidence:** The book concludes by encouraging you to embrace menopause as a new beginning. It equips you with the knowledge and confidence needed to navigate this stage of life with grace and self-assuredness.

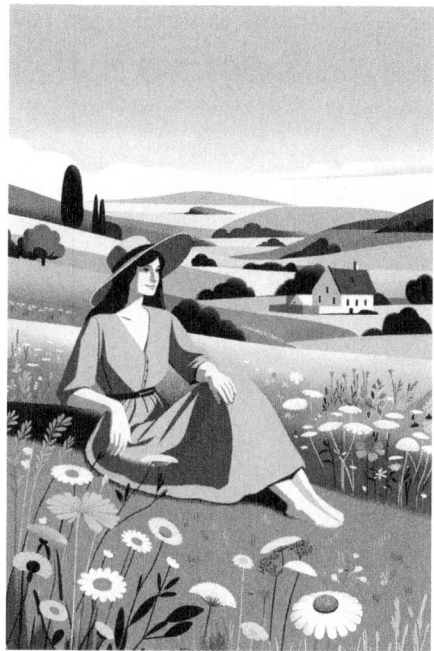

Are you ready to take charge of your menopausal journey and discover the path to a healthier, happier you? If you want to navigate menopause with grace, *The Ultimate Guide to Menopause* is your go-to resource for:

- **A holistic approach:** This book offers a unique perspective by addressing not only the physical symptoms but also the emotional, spiritual, and relational aspects of menopause. I believe true empowerment during this phase comes from a well-rounded approach.
- **Cutting-edge information:** Menopause can be overwhelming, but this book provides the latest research and evidence-based information to help you make informed decisions and effectively manage this phase of your life.
- **Actionable solutions:** Within these pages, we'll go beyond theory. This book equips you with practical tools,

including tailored workouts, nutrition plans, and mindfulness practices that you can immediately integrate into your life.

In a world overloaded with information, this book stands out as your clear, actionable, and holistic guide to managing menopause. It's the right book for you if you want to embrace this phase of your life with confidence and vitality.

Don't wait any longer; it's time to take control and make this transition your own. *The Ultimate Guide to Menopause* will help you ease the physical and emotional transitions that menopause brings, and together, we'll navigate this phase with strength, wisdom, and a sense of community. We will journey through the 7-Component BALANCE Framework for fighting symptoms of menopause and fostering well-being:

- **B**etter symptom management
- **A**dopting healthy nutrition
- **L**iving actively
- **A**chieving inner peace and resilience
- **N**urturing empowerment
- **C**ultivating relationships
- **E**mbracing menopause with confidence

So, let's explore the strategies in this comprehensive guidebook to manage your menopausal symptoms and changes and embark on this empowering and stress-relieving journey together.

1

UNDERSTANDING MENOPAUSE

From fragile bones, pounding joints, no desire to be intimate, a foggy brain, and vaginal discomfort to problems sleeping, experiencing intense emotions, going from happy to angry in less than 60 seconds, and drowning in the sweat of your angry hot flashes, each woman's experience differs. What do we have in common? The uncertainty and inconvenience that menopause brings to our lives.

Yes, we may agree that none of us experience menopause in the same way, but one thing's for sure: Sharing our stories with each other is useful, inspirational, and empowering. If I had a dollar for every time someone has asked what menopause is, I'd be filthy rich. However, what menopause really entails is a subject people hardly ever talk about, so it's no surprise that so many women are confused about what it is and whether they're going through it or not. To recognize whether your menopausal phase has truly started, you need to understand what exactly menopause is.

MENOPAUSE AS A NATURAL LIFE STAGE

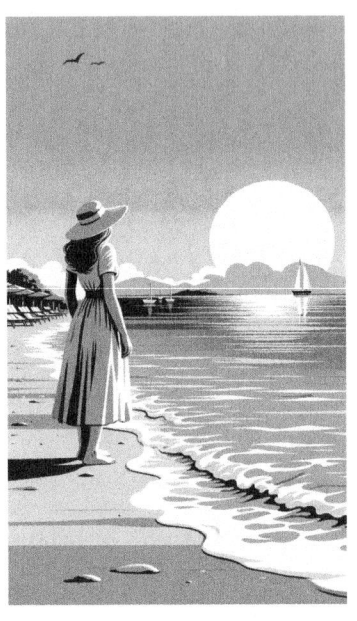

Menopause, a natural and inevitable life stage, marks the end of your reproductive years, accompanied by a rainbow of experiences as diverse as you—the woman who will undergo this transformative process. It's important to know that menopause is a natural part of your journey as a woman, and it's not a disease or something you need to hide or be embarrassed about.

While estrogen depletion during menopause is linked to many conditions like heart disease and osteoporosis, understanding this transition allows you to proactively manage symptoms and other conditions that may accompany your menopause. Your personal health status, lifestyle choices, and other influences like your genetics may have a great influence on your quality of life during your menopausal life stage.

I'd like you to know that, despite the associated challenges you may be facing, effective treatments exist for conditions related to estrogen depletion.

Applying holistic care during this transformative phase in your life will empower you and help you overcome your challenges one day at a time.

What Is Premenopause?

Premenopause refers to the phase in your life that happens from the start of your first period up until perimenopause, which is then followed by full-on menopause. During the premenopausal stage, you likely won't experience any symptoms related to menopause as these will only start in the perimenopausal phase (Pugle, 2021). It's important to note that premenopause can vary in duration for each female. Some women begin experiencing perimenopause and related symptoms much earlier than others.

What exactly is the difference between perimenopause and premenopause? I know, all these terms can get pretty confusing. Perimenopause and premenopause are terms that are often used interchangeably, but they actually refer to different phases in a woman's reproductive life. So let's take a look at the differences (Nall, 2023a):

- **Premenopause (long before menopause):** This is the phase before perimenopause, from when you start menstruating as a young woman up to when your reproductive hormones begin to decline. It is marked by hormonal shifts and occasional irregularities in the menstrual cycle. However, you will still have your period regularly and will likely not experience any harsh symptoms unless you have another female-related condition.
- **Perimenopause (just before menopause):** Usually the years right before menopause are called "perimenopause." This is the time when your body goes through more intense hormonal changes and prepares your body for the end of your reproductive years. In the perimenopause stage, the production of estrogen by your ovaries decreases

(yup, your hormones start to run empty), leading to potential irregularities in your menstrual cycle. You may experience various symptoms such as emotional fluctuations, insomnia, sudden body heat, or excessive sweating during the night—another reason you won't get enough sleep! Perimenopause can start several years before menopause (WebMD Editorial Contributors, n.d.-e).

- **The crossover into menopause consists of two stages:**

  - **Beginning:** During the first stage of perimenopause, changes in the duration and strength of menstruation happen, and there may be abrupt spikes in estrogen levels (*Menopause*, 2022). Perimenopause typically starts in the early 40s but can begin in some women's 30s (Mayo Clinic Staff, 2023c).
  - **Mature:** The more mature stage of perimenopause usually occurs in a woman's late 40s to early 50s. During this stage, women start missing periods until they eventually stop altogether. Around six months prior to menopause, there is a notable decline in estrogen levels, resulting in menopausal symptoms that can continue for a duration ranging from six months to five years or more after menopause begins (*Menopause*, 2022).

What Is Menopause?

Menopause happens when your ovarian follicular activity declines, reducing the estrogen levels in your bloodstream (World Health Organization, 2022). Yup, your ovaries are slowing down.

Natural menopause is officially recognized when a woman doesn't menstruate for 12 uninterrupted cycles without any other identifiable reasons. Premature menopause happens in some women prior to the age of 40. It can be caused by chromosomal anomalies, diseases affecting the immune system, or other unknown elements (World Health Organization, 2022).

Establishing when menopause will knock on your door is challenging, to say the least. Remember, some genetic, health-related, or environmental, socioeconomic, and cultural influences may play a role in when menopause will start for a specific person (World Health Organization, 2022).

Menopause can also be kick-started by medical therapies, such as radiotherapy, or as a side-effect of surgical procedures like oophorectomy, a procedure where one or both of a woman's ovaries are removed (Mayo Clinic Staff, 2022a). Some women may stop menstruating before reaching menopause due to specific medications like birth control pills, and they may also be affected by other symptoms connected to menopause (World Health Organization, 2022)

The Final Stage: Postmenopause

Congratulations! If you are in the category of women who have survived more than a year without a period, you may start to enter the postmenopausal stage (Rose, 2023). But don't get excited too soon—many women in the final stage still struggle with symptoms caused by menopause. And unfortunately, some women may suffer from long-term conditions that result from menopause, such as heart conditions.

No matter where you are in your menopause journey, your body has already gone through changes, is currently going through changes, and will keep changing for the rest of your life. Embracing these changes can be tough, and that's exactly why I have written this book—to help you shift your perspective and make these changes more manageable for you.

THE IMPORTANCE OF SELF-CARE IN THE PREMENOPAUSAL PHASE

Considering the hormonal fluctuations and diverse symptoms associated with menopause, taking care of yourself during the premenopausal phase is crucial for your well-being. Engaging in self-care practices can help you effectively navigate these changes and foster a healthier lifestyle. Regular exercise can enhance your overall wellness by helping you control your weight and increase your strength.

Additionally, self-care can help you manage your mental and emotional health, reduce any feelings of anxiety you might be experiencing, and help you accept yourself during this natural stage of life.

As a woman, it's essential to prioritize self-care during the premenopausal phase to support your wellness and make your transitions to the perimenopausal and postmenopausal periods less shaky. If we neglect self-care during premenopause, our bodies will face greater challenges in maintaining balance amid the regular hormonal fluctuations.

Keep in mind that the longer you withhold this support from your body, the more severe these menopausal symptoms can become.

Understanding the Concept of Balance and Its Connection to Self-Care

Can you recall your high school biology class? Do you remember the term "homeostasis"? Homeostasis pertains to the various processes employed by living organisms to uphold relatively consistent circumstances crucial for their existence, such as a consistent body temperature (Rodolfo, 2000).

Our bodies constantly strive to achieve and sustain homeostasis, which is the state of equilibrium and balance across numerous bodily systems.

To illustrate, your body strives to keep a constant temperature of 98 °F (*Self-Care in Perimenopause*, n.d.). Hormone changes in menopause make it difficult for your body to regulate its temperature. This causes the most commonly recognized signs of menopause—hot flashes and night sweats.

As our final batch of eggs is released, the delicate system that orchestrates our monthly cycles undergoes a transformation. Any part of our body that possesses receivers for estrogen and progesterone—the hormones that experience the most significant changes—can become a bit chaotic to manage! This transformation unleashes a whirlwind of hormonal surprises, affecting various aspects of our bodies.

Our human vessels need our support, especially now, to find and maintain a balance and keep the ship sailing safely in the water. That's where self-care plays a role, becoming a necessity rather than a choice.

If you're concerned that embracing this life stage implies that you are getting older and your life is over, rest assured, that's not what it means. This quote sums it up accurately: "Self-care is not an indulgence. It's a discipline" (Forman, 2017). We can recognize that self-care is, indeed, a job. It's an important task that will empower you to endure and flourish in this stage of your life.

Finding solace in our minds may not always come easily, but embracing acceptance as a daily practice can help ease the burden of stress and bring us closer to a sense of inner balance—the equilibrium our bodies constantly yearn for.

Embrace perimenopause as an opportunity for self-care and personal growth. It's the best gift you can choose to give yourself.

YOUR BODY CHANGING BECAUSE OF MENOPAUSE

As I mentioned earlier, during menopause, dynamic hormonal changes take place in the female body because of the decline in ovarian function (Su & Freeman, 2009). Let's unpack the science behind it and figure out why you are experiencing certain symptoms.

The key hormones measured in menopause include anti-Mullerian hormone (AMH), estradiol estrogen, inhibin B, and follicle-stimulating hormone (FSH). These hormones experience changes throughout the menopausal transition, with AMH, inhibin B, and estrogen levels declining and FSH levels growing (Su & Freeman, 2009). Interestingly, the levels of estrogen either remain stable or exhibit a tendency to increase until the transition begins, whereafter it declines rapidly (Burger et al., 2002).

So, what exactly happens when estrogen undergoes fluctuations or decreases during perimenopause? Because estrogen helps pump enough blood to your vagina and keeps it moist and intact, a decrease in estrogen impacts your sexual function by causing vaginal dryness. Your sex life is also implicitly affected by intrusive and tiring symptoms such as night sweats and hot flashes. (NAMS, n.d.-a).

Other symptoms related to hormonal changes during menopause may include insomnia, emotional fluctuations, and changes in your sex drive (*Menopause*, 2022).

Another occurrence is the decrease in size of your follicle pool, resulting in a decrease in inhibin B levels and an increase in FSH levels, indicating a reduction in inhibin control. The removal of inhibin's control over FSH release seems to be the initial hormonal change that causes a shorter menstrual cycle and some of the hormonal fluctuations experienced during the later reproductive years (Sowers et al., 2008). This may also be connected to the decrease in fertility that occurs as you age reproductively (Hurwitz & Santoro, 2004).

Enough science lessons for now. Let's look a bit deeper at some of the day-to-day signs and symptoms that happen during menopause.

Signs and Symptoms Explained

Many tissues within the female body possess numerous estrogen receivers, and a decline in estrogen levels can directly impact various organs. The signs and symptoms of menopause can manifest at different stages, including early, intermediate, or late stages.

- **Your menstrual cycle changing:** At first, your monthly period will become more irregular, then it will become shorter and eventually go away completely. You will encounter more or even less bleeding than usual, and sporadic spotting may occur. If a period is skipped, you need to confirm that you are not pregnant. If you're not, the absence of your period could suggest the start of menopause. If you do have spotting occurring when you haven't seen a monthly period for 12 months in a row, it's advisable to consult your doctor to ensure that you don't have any potentially harmful illnesses (Saljoughian, 2018).

- **A dry vagina:** Once your body produces less progesterone and estrogen, it may lead to a dry vagina. This may affect the natural moisture that lines your vaginal walls. Your vagina may dry out at any age, but this often becomes a bigger issue when you're experiencing menopause. The lower estrogen levels during menopause can bring on biological shifts. This is when you lose your interest in having intercourse. Try to remember that when you have intercourse, it promotes blood moving to your vagina, helping to maintain lubrication and potentially preventing the thinning of your vagina.

- **Hot flashes:** A hot flash is an unexpected sensation of heat, like a wave of warmth, that occurs throughout your body, although some women may only experience it in their upper extremities. When you encounter a hot flash, your face and neck may become red, and you may feel flushed or sweaty. Many women have hot flashes for approximately one to two years following their last period. The intensity of a hot flash can vary from moderate to intense, and in some cases, it may even disrupt your sleep. A standard hot flash usually lasts from 30 seconds to 10 minutes (*What Is Menopause?*, n.d.). While hot flashes may persist after menopause, they generally become less intense over time (Freeman et al., 2014).

- **Itching in the vulvar area and vaginal atrophy:** Has intercourse become a distressing and unpleasant experience? Do you feel like you need to go to the bathroom the whole time? Does your vagina feel dry during sex? On top of this, are you having trouble with a tingling, itchy vulva? Dryness and itching can be relieved by using a water-based lubricant or vaginal moisturizer. The thinning of your vaginal lining can cause it to become infected, creating great discomfort. If treatment with lubricants or moisturizers doesn't do the trick, you may opt for a vaginal estrogen treatment (Saljoughian, 2018).

- **Inflammation of your urinary tract:** A decrease in estrogen and disruptions in your urinary tract can increase your susceptibility to infections during menopause. Symptoms such as a burning feeling and an unstoppable need to urinate may indicate that your urinary tract is inflamed. If this is the case, you need to visit your doctor, who is likely to prescribe antibiotics (Saljoughian, 2018).

- **Incontinence and bladder weakness:** While in your menopausal period, the decrease in estrogen levels can result in incontinence and weakened bladder function. This occurs when your pelvic muscles and tissues, which support the bladder and urethra, become weaker, and unplanned urine seeping may occur, such as unexpected seeping when you cough. Menopause can lead to various types of urinary incontinence. Stress incontinence happens when the muscles of the bladder and urethra become weak. Urge incontinence occurs when the bladder muscles become overactive. Mixed urinary incontinence is a mix of urinary incontinence symptoms along with an overactive bladder (Kołodyńska et al., 2019). Other factors —like pregnancy, childbirth, being overweight, pelvic organ prolapse, and certain health conditions such as diabetes, stroke, Parkinson's disease, and multiple sclerosis —can also contribute to these problems. Treatment options include exercises to improve your bladder function, including making the muscles in the pelvic floor stronger through Kegel exercises, as well as getting the right medication and adapting your diet to support your bladder health. You can also visit a urologist and discuss specific options for surgery if the problem becomes unbearable (*Menopause Incontinence*, n.d.).

- **Changing moods:** Mood symptoms can be a challenging aspect of menopause. If you are in the middle of menopause, you may be having unpredictable moods, including being anxious, emotional despair and disinterest, getting easily agitated, having trouble focusing, showcasing hostile behavior, frequently feeling extremely tense, and being tired nonstop (Saljoughian, 2018). While there may be other factors that can contribute to you not feeling like yourself, you might be surprised to hear that these signs are typical during menopause. The good news is that there are ways to control your moods. Adjustments in your lifestyle, such as better managing your stress and adopting relaxation techniques, such as meditation, deep breathing, Tai Chi, and yoga, can positively impact and help you start feeling like yourself again in no time.

- **Skin and hair changes***:* As time goes by, the natural aging process can bring about noticeable changes. When you lose collagen and fatty tissue, your skin may become dryer and thinner than ever before. This can also impact the suppleness and moistness of the skin surrounding your vagina. Lower estrogen levels might accelerate hair loss or make your hair feel parched and fragile. Chemical hair treatments may exacerbate the issue (Saljoughian, 2018).

- **Osteoporosis***:* After menopause, your body has less estrogen, and the breakdown of bones happens faster than the development of new bone mass in your body. When this happens, it leads to a condition called "osteoporosis." Premature menopause before the age of 45 or prolonged reduced hormone levels can result in a decline in bone density. Osteoporosis may not have apparent signs until the bones weaken, leading to fractures or collapsed vertebrae. Aside from menopause, other things may increase your chances of getting osteoporosis. Your age, bone structure, ethnicity, body weight, gender, and even your family medical history may all have an influence (Saljoughian, 2018). Do you feel like you're getting shorter as you age? You just might be right. In postmenopausal women, a compressed vertebra can cause back discomfort, changes in spinal alignment, and height reduction. Hormone therapy during menopause is believed to help prevent or slow down the rate of bone density loss, especially in premature menopause (*Menopause and Osteoporosis*, n.d.).

- **Cardiovascular problems:** The occurrence of cardiovascular disease rises after menopause. Women who have gone through menopause have a higher chance of developing coronary heart disease in comparison to women who haven't reached menopause yet. This increased risk may be due to a decrease in estrogen levels in postmenopausal women (Ryczkowska et al., 2023). Estrogen may favorably impact the inner layer of your artery wall, promoting flexibility and allowing for proper blood flow. Regardless of its benefits, the American Heart Association advises against using postmenopausal hormone therapy to lessen the occurrence of coronary heart disease or stroke, as it may not be effective (American Heart Association Editorial Staff, n.d.).
- **Decreased sex drive:** During menopause, you may find that you are less interested in sex. This can be caused by your hormones being out of whack, low testosterone levels, or other menopausal symptoms like constantly

being tired, sleep changes, experiencing a dry vagina, feeling depressed or grumpy (*Common Symptoms*, 2014).

- **Night sweats and cold flashes:** Night sweats are basically hot flashes that happen while you're sleeping. They raise your body temperature quickly, leading to heavy sweating (Nadeem, 2023). Are you ever awakened to find yourself in pajamas that are drenched in sweat? Yup, that's most likely night sweats, but also check that your room isn't too warm. Please don't take it lightly, as night sweats may also indicate more serious conditions that should be checked out (Stöppler, n.d.). Some women may experience sudden chills or cold flashes, too. Sometimes it happens after hot flashes, and you will feel cold and your body shivering.

- **Increased weight and slowed metabolism:** Menopause can cause your weight to increase and make your metabolism slower because of a decrease in muscle mass, which means fewer calories are getting burned. Lower estrogen levels might also affect how fat is distributed in your body, leading to more abdominal fat and weight increases (*Symptoms*, n.d.).

- **Joint and muscle stiffness and pains:** Arthralgia refers to joints that frequently feel painful. This is a general symptom of menopause, impeding areas such as the hips, hands, shoulders, knees, neck, and fingers (Physiopedia Contributors, n.d.). The loss of estrogen during menopause can impact joints and connective tissue, resulting in general muscle cramps, pains, and stiffness (Nadeem, 2023).

- **Headaches:** You may experience headaches during menopause due to changes in estrogen levels, including a decrease in estrogen around the time of your menstrual cycle. Right at the start of your menopause, these headaches may be the worst (*Common Symptoms*, 2014). It's hard to tell you exactly why you're having these incidents as it can be a multitude of things, such as too little sleep, dehydration, constant stress, too much sugar intake, and even eating certain foods and spices that are bad for your health. Write down exactly when these happen, as it may form a pattern that your doctor can interpret to make a diagnosis.

- **Heart palpitations:** During menopause, you may feel your heart racing, have an uncomfortable or irregular heartbeat, or sense a flip-flopping in your chest (Nadeem, 2023). The reason behind these palpitations is the decrease in estrogen levels that occurs during menopause. It's important to note that this change in hormone levels can increase the risk of heart palpitations.

- **Constantly feeling tired:** Menopause can be tiring—for real! During this stage, many women experience fatigue due to hormonal changes and disrupted sleep patterns. Hormonal fluctuations, particularly a decrease in estrogen, can cause frequent waking during the night, making it difficult for you to get consistent quality sleep. Fatigue during menopause not only affects your energy levels but also your mental and emotional wellness, leading to edginess, anxiety, and even depression. Fortunately, there are effective treatments available to manage menopause fatigue. Lifestyle adjustments such as regular exercise, staying hydrated, and prioritizing good sleep habits can help alleviate your fatigue symptoms. Hormone therapy is another option that can improve your sleep quality and boost your energy levels (WebMD Editorial Contributors, n.d.-d).

- **Sleep disruptions:** Menopause can disturb your sleep, making it difficult to fall asleep or stay asleep. You might wake up earlier than you planned and struggle to sleep again. Not only that, you may have to go to the bathroom, and you are sweating like a hot horse! To enhance your sleep, it can be helpful to practice relaxation and breathing techniques. Engaging in activities like taking a bath, reading, or listening to soothing music before bedtime can promote relaxation. Moreover, maintaining a regular exercise routine during the day is crucial. Establishing a consistent bedtime routine, creating a cool sleeping environment, and avoiding sleep-disrupting substances like caffeine, alcohol, or chocolate can all contribute to bettering the quality of your sleep (*Common Symptoms*, 2014).

- **Brain fog:** Have you ever experienced brain fog? It's like your thoughts are hiding from you! During menopause, low estrogen levels, a lack of sleep, and stress can all cause memory issues and brain fog, affecting your ability to remember, your concentration, and your decision-making skills (Ask the Doctors, 2021). But fear not! You can combat this foggy situation with regular exercise, meditation, and mindfulness to reduce stress and anxiety. Keep your brain and body active to prevent memory loss during menopause. Let's outsmart that brain fog together (*How to Combat Menopausal Brain Fog,* 2022)!

It's important to know that there might be other symptoms related to menopause that are not listed above, although I tried to be as thorough as possible! For other symptoms, please consult your doctor. To keep a symptom checklist, use the symptom checker in the Bonus chapter of this book.

THE 7-COMPONENT BALANCE FRAMEWORK FOR MENOPAUSE

The 7-Component BALANCE Framework for Menopause is a holistic approach with seven easy steps to tackle symptoms of menopause head-on and foster your well-being. The framework includes the following components:

- **B**etter symptom management
- **A**dopting healthy nutrition
- **L**iving actively
- **A**chieving inner peace and resilience
- **N**urturing empowerment
- **C**ultivating relationships
- **E**mbracing menopause with confidence

The 7-Component BALANCE Framework for Menopause delves into a broad variety of topics, including strategies to address post-menopausal hormonal imbalances, maintaining a healthy weight, following a balanced diet that incorporates a variety of nutrient-rich foods, exercising regularly, and keeping your gut healthy (EliteCare Health Centers, 2023). Vasomotor symptoms (VMS) are the result of the contraction and expansion of your blood vessels (Nall, 2023b). For managing VMS, like night sweats and hot flashes, hormone therapy has been noted as highly effective (Mayo Clinic Staff, 2023a). We will discuss this alongside nonhormonal alternatives, such as venlafaxine, citalopram, gabapentin, and paroxetine, which have shown a reduction in symptom frequency (Crandall et al., 2023).

We will talk about making changes to your diet to help with menopausal symptoms. This includes adding foods that are rich in calcium, whole grains, vegetables, fruits, healthy fats, foods with phytoestrogens, and good sources of protein. We will also discuss steering clear of certain foods, like added sugars, which may help to stop weight gain, alleviate hot flashes, and better your sleep (Groves, 2023).

The framework will also encompass different solutions for managing menopausal symptoms, such as calming practices, stress management, eating well, engaging in daily physical activity, and exploring hormone therapies (NAMS, n.d.-b).

Chapter 1 gave you the lowdown on what menopause is all about, breaking down the nitty-gritty and what factors play into it. Now, let's switch gears to Chapter 2, where we'll tackle the first component of the 7-Component BALANCE Framework and talk about ways to make dealing with your menopause symptoms a bit easier. We'll be diving into practical tips and tricks, from lifestyle changes to possible medical solutions, all aimed at helping women go through this phase with a bit more comfort and ease.

2

BETTER SYMPTOM MANAGEMENT

M y friend Jenna had quite an unpleasant time when she experienced menopause alongside her thyroid disease. After receiving medical help for her overactive thyroid, she depended on medication to replace her thyroid hormone function. The real challenge came when Jenna's menopause started, leaving her confused about which symptoms were thyroid issues and which were related to her menopause.

Jenna couldn't cope with untimely hot flashes anymore. Despite successfully managing her thyroid condition, the worsening of her menopausal symptoms prompted her to find medical support. Her doctor recommended a trial of hormone replacement therapy (HRT), which involved a combination of estrogen and proges-terone treatment taken in a specific sequence. Thankfully, the HRT effectively relieved her menopausal symptoms. However, it did not fully resolve the ongoing concerns about her thyroid levels.

The connection between menopause and thyroid function became more noticeable when Jenna's thyroid stimulating hormone (TSH) levels started to decrease during this time. It became clear that managing both conditions would be a total headache, requiring careful adjustments to her chronic thyroid medicine by her endocrinologist. Following each adjustment, her blood was retested after six weeks, and the medicine was adjusted again. This continued until her thyroid levels returned to the normal range, which took about 12 months.

As you can see from Jenna's experience, having other chronic conditions can impact menopause and vice versa. Her story highlights the importance of finding the right balance of hormones and the need for personalized care to address the unique aspects of both menopause and other disorders. Jenna was lucky to have a doctor who followed the right approach to treat her. Many women struggle endlessly with finding the right way to manage their continuous symptoms.

This chapter focuses on the first part of the 7-Component BALANCE Framework, which is (B): Better symptom management. Here, we'll discuss the common symptoms experienced during menopause, identify warning signs that may require medical attention, and provide a wide range of methods to help you find relief. These methods include traditional Western medical solutions as well as complementary and alternative therapies.

A holistic approach to finding the right diagnosis and managing your menopause symptoms involves making changes in your lifestyle, like starting and sticking to a healthy diet, engaging in regular exercise, and implementing effective stress management techniques. My goal is to support you in managing your symptoms effectively. Let's talk about some options you have when it comes to tackling menopausal symptoms.

WESTERN MEDICAL SOLUTIONS

There are medical treatments available to support you when you're experiencing menopause: hormone replacement therapy (HRT)—whether estrogen on its own or a combined therapy with progestogen, which is the synthetic hormone designed to replicate the results of progesterone in the body, and, if needed, the use of testosterone (Wilkinson, n.d.).

HRT entails taking estrogen to renew your body's depleted levels when you are experiencing menopause. Doing so helps alleviate many of the symptoms you may be facing, like struggling to get a good night's rest, forgetting things, hot flushing, a dry vagina, moodiness, and painful joints.

If your womb is still intact, taking progestogen alongside estrogen is important to protect yourself from diseases like cancer and other symptoms such as unexpected bleeding. When you are already receiving HRT but are also struggling with a decreased libido that doesn't improve, the doctor may consider prescribing some testosterone to assist you (NHS, n.d.-c).

I want to say this early on: This book is here to assist you on your journey, inform you about menopause, share what other women have found to work, and tell you where you can find help. I am not providing you with any medical advice whatsoever. It's important to have a conversation with your healthcare provider, who can provide personalized treatment options based on your specific needs and medical history, and to attend regular checkups to ensure that the treatment is effective and monitor any potential side effects or changes in your symptoms.

Although HRT is seen as safe and effective for most women, it can be dangerous in some cases. These dangers may include blood clotting events, breast cancer, strokes, and heart disease (*Hormone Replacement Therapy [HRT]*, 2022). Your susceptibility to these risks may depend on a variety of factors. Therefore, I repeat, you need to consult with your doctor when considering HRT. They will consider your individual circumstances, risks, and personal treatment goals.

Different Kinds of Hormone Therapy for Menopause

Different types of HRT may help if you experience intense menopausal symptoms. Let's talk about the differences:

- **Estrogen replacement therapy (ERT):** ERT uses estrogen to replace the natural amount of estrogen in the body during menopause. Sufficient estrogen equals healthy bones (*Hormone Replacement Therapy [HRT]*, 2022). Estrogen can be given through implants or suppositories, sprays, skin patches, creams, gels, or tablets (NHS, n.d.-c).

  - **Vaginal estrogen** is used to help with vaginal dryness and discomfort during intercourse and is considered to be a highly effective low-dose treatment. It is available in a cream, gel, vaginal ring or tablet, or an intrauterine device (IUD) like a Mirena. It is a long-term treatment option as it only releases small quantities of estrogen into the bloodstream. Estrogen in lower doses is not believed to raise the risk of stroke, breast cancer, or heart attacks (Santen & Loprinzi, 2023).
  - **Estrogen-only HRT** is commonly utilized by women who have undergone a hysterectomy (NHS, n.d.-c). It involves taking estrogen alone as there is no need for progestogen if your womb has been removed.

- **Combined hormone replacement therapy:** Both estrogen and progestogen are taken with this type of HRT. When you are receiving estrogen and haven't undergone a hysterectomy, it's important that you also consider taking progestogen. Estrogen may thicken your womb's lining, which could result in other health issues, like unexpected bleeding. Progestogen can be given in patches, by drinking dissolvable tablets, or as part of a combined patch along with estrogen.
- **Testosterone therapy:** Testosterone, in a gel form, may be offered if low libido persists despite HRT (NHS, n.d.-c).
- **Combined HRT with testosterone:** This medication is comparable to combined HRT (estrogen and progestogen) but also includes testosterone. It is consumed orally and is an appropriate treatment option to consider if your most recent period occurred over a year ago. It is used to treat postmenopausal osteoporosis, and it helps with mood problems and hot flashes. (NHS, n.d.-c; *Types of Hormone Therapy*, n.d.).

Adverse Reactions of HRT

Here are some examples of the side effects that may result from HRT (*Types of Hormone Therapy*, n.d.):

- queasiness and vomiting
- irregular bleeding
- tenderness in your breasts
- mood changes
- frequent headaches
- retaining water in your body
- swelling in the abdomen (distension)

If you observe any of these reactions, you need to inform your doctor right away. Adjusting the dosage or switching to a different type of HRT might be options that can alleviate these effects. Never modify your dosage or discontinue HRT without consulting your doctor.

NONHORMONAL SOLUTIONS FOR MENOPAUSE

Nonhormonal medications can be an effective option for managing hot flashes and mood symptoms during menopause. These medications may not make you the life of the party, but they can certainly help cool down those hot flashes and bring some comfort! Here are some examples of these medications:

- **Selective serotonin reuptake inhibitors (SSRIs):** Paxil (active ingredient paroxetine) is an SSRI known for its efficacy in managing hot flushing. Other SSRIs, such as Celexa (active ingredient citalopram) and Prozac (active ingredient fluoxetine) may also help alleviate it (Merz, 2017; Santen & Loprinzi, 2023).
- **Serotonin-norepinephrine reuptake inhibitors (SNRIs):** Medications such as Effexor (active ingredient venlafaxine) can help manage hot flushing and mood symptoms (Merz, 2017).
- **Clonidine:** This blood pressure medication can be used to help lessen those angry hot flashes (*Types of Hormone Therapy*, n.d.).
- **Gabapentin:** Normally prescribed for seizures, it can help alleviate those pesky hot flashes too (*Types of Hormone Therapy*, n.d.).
- **Nonhormonal treatments for vaginal dryness:** This involves two effective approaches—moisturizers and lubricants. Vaginal moisturizers stick to or get absorbed by

the tissue in the vagina, continuously alleviating your pain, discomfort, and itching. Different than lubricants, moisturizers are designed to be applied frequently. Lubricants are liquids or gels made from water or silicone, and they help lessen resistance during sexual activity. You can use them right before having sex, but they won't provide long-term comfort (Harvard Health Publishing, n.d.; Merz, 2017).

I encourage you to talk to your doctor to find the right nonhormonal treatment that fits your needs and personal medical history. Ask your doctor as many questions as you need about the pros and cons of these different options.

LIFESTYLE CHANGES

Lifestyle changes can be a successful way to manage your menopause symptoms. If you are experiencing symptoms like angry heat flashes, trouble sleeping, and moods that are out of whack, being physically active and following a nutritious eating plan may comfort you. If you smoke, you should stop because it can make your hot flushing happen more often, and it can become more intense (Balzer, 2021).

Make your sleeping environment as comfortable as possible, and when you get dressed, be mindful to wear fabrics that are not too warm.

To manage night sweats and hot flashes, try avoiding stimuli like caffeine and hot, richly flavored foods. Don't be discouraged from having your morning cup (I know you may need it!), but it's best to avoid these stimuli after midday. Women who have excess weight often feel more discomfort from hot flashes than women whose weight is in the normal range. Losing weight can lessen the intensity of hot flushing and has many other benefits for your health (*Hot Flashes: What Can I Do?*, n.d.). To help you improve your lifestyle choices, we will talk more about diet, weight loss, and exercise in Chapters 3 and 4.

MIND-BODY APPROACHES

Consider trying cognitive-behavioral therapy (CBT), which consists of talking therapy, regulated breathing, and relaxation activities like yoga, Tai Chi, and meditation to help you deal with stress. CBT can also help you sleep better and improve your mood and overall wellness. Other techniques like hypnosis, acupuncture, and aromatherapy may help manage menopausal symptoms (Johnson et al., 2019). Remember, you have the power to take control of your health and find relief from hot flashes! We'll talk in greater detail about yoga and Tai Chi in Chapter 4, but let's first talk about CBT and other techniques.

Cognitive-Behavioral Therapy

Cognitive-behavioral therapy (CBT) can be really helpful for managing menopause symptoms like low mood, anxiety, and sleep problems. With CBT, you'll explore the connections between your thoughts, emotions, physical reactions, and behaviors. It's a short therapy lasting up to six consultations that zooms in on proactive ways to manage your problems and develop new coping mechanisms (Hunter & Chilcot, 2021). If you want to read up some more on this, the MENOS CBT protocol has been suggested as a nonhormonal treatment for menopausal symptoms (The North American Menopause Society, 2015).

CBT can help you manage hot flashes, reduce stress, and improve your sleep quality. It's great for improving your overall quality of life. CBT may be sufficient with or without additional assistance. CBT is also suggested for treating anxiety and depression during your menopause and postmenopausal phases (Hunter, n.d.).

Hypnosis

If sleepless nights aren't enough, you may also be experiencing brain fog throughout the day. Who said mommy-brain ends after pregnancy? Whatever, they lied! Did you know that hypnosis is a helpful treatment for managing menopause symptoms? When you enter a focused state of concentration through hypnosis, it helps you change any anxious thoughts or behaviors you may have rehearsed into more flexible thoughts and behaviors. By focusing on cooling imagery during hypnosis, you can gain greater control over the frequency and severity of your angry hot flashes (Jack, 2020).

Hypnosis has demonstrated a remarkable ability to lessen hot flushing by more than 70%, proving its effectiveness comparable to HRT for symptom management (Elkins et al., 2013). Not only that, but hypnosis can also better your sleep quality and lessen anxiety.

Hypnosis is a safe, relaxing, and noninvasive therapy that can be used alongside other treatments to manage your menopause symptoms. If you're interested in trying self-hypnosis, it's a great method for improving sleep in menopausal women, whether you decide to do it virtually or in person (Otte et al., 2020).

Below are three techniques to practice (Jack, 2020):

- Start off with a preferred breathing technique or some meditation to help you relax. Alternatively, envision inhaling a cool, silvery light through your nose, allowing it to flow throughout your body as you breathe out. Repeat this process while affirming, "I'm relaxed now." In this tranquil state, visualize the most delightful cooling sensation for you, such as walking with your toes in the sand on the beach. The next time you feel a hot flash starting, concentrate on this image and sensation to help you relax.

- Envision how you wish to feel a few months from now. While closing your eyes, imagine a picture with all the feelings, smells, and sounds you would like your future self to experience. Think of the steps needed to manifest this future self. It may involve clarifying your life goals, saving some money, decluttering your house, incorporating exercise like yoga, or practicing more self-care. Revisit this image regularly to keep yourself motivated to implement positive life changes.

- Visualize a clock that ranges from 0 to 10, the lowest representing cool comfort and the highest extreme heat. Determine your current position on this clock, then experiment with turning the cursor upward and downward. Feel your body temperature rise as you turn the cursor higher and decrease as you lower it. Repeat this a few times before setting it to where you feel most comfortable. Practice this control exercise often so that when a hot flash comes on, you can use it to regulate your body heat.

Meditation, Mindfulness, and Relaxation

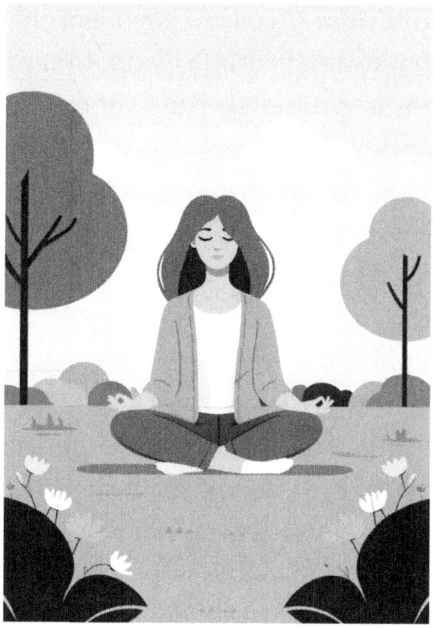

Meditate your way through menopause and kick symptoms like stress, anxiety, irritability, depression, hot flashes, and insomnia in the butt. Here's why you should try meditating:

- **Mindfulness and menopause:** When you practice mindfulness, a form of meditation that focuses on the moment you're in, it can help alleviate symptoms like anxiety, agitation, stress, night sweats, depression, and hot flashes (*Does Mindfulness Help With Menopause?*, 2023).
- **Impact on blood chemistry:** Did you know that practicing activities like yoga, Tai Chi, and meditation can have a positive impact on women's health during menopause? These mind-body therapies may help lessen menopausal symptoms and even influence blood chemistry, so including these practices in your routine

could make a difference in how you feel overall (Sung et al., 2020).

- **Bedtime meditation:** If you are having problems falling asleep, incorporating a bedtime meditation practice can train your body and mind for rest (Abramson, 2022).

Something else that's worth trying to improve your wellness and alleviate your menopausal symptoms are relaxation techniques and breathing exercises. Here are some specific examples, but make sure to search for more online (Jones, 2023; WebMD Editorial Contributors, n.d.-b):

- **Timed breathing:** Inhale slowly, allowing your chest to expand for 5 seconds. Then exhale for 5 seconds. Practice these steps for 10 minutes twice daily or for 5 minutes when you are having a hot flash.
- **Extensive focused breathing:** Breathe extensively into your abdomen, filling it with air. Then exhale slowly.
- **Envisioned breathing:** While taking slow breaths, visualize relaxation entering your body and tension leaving it.
- **Progressive muscle relaxation:** Carefully stress and then relax each muscle group, but be sure to avoid causing yourself any discomfort in the process. Start slowly from your head, moving down to your toes to promote overall relaxation.

These techniques work by regulating your oxygen intake and slowing your heart rate, reducing hot flashes and other menopausal symptoms.

COMPLEMENTARY AND ALTERNATIVE REMEDIES

Although menopause is the friend you did not choose, it's also the friend that will be by your side for quite a long time. You might as well embrace it. Make sure to manage it in your favor. By now, you may be wondering if there are any natural remedies to help you survive and thrive on your journey with menopause. The great news is the answer is yes, yes, and yes!

Many women who prefer alternative options or cannot use HRT often look for complementary remedies to manage their menopause symptoms. Keep in mind that while some women may find these remedies helpful, the evidence of their effectiveness varies. As always, you should consult with a healthcare provider before trying any new treatments.

Acupuncture

You may find acupuncture to be a supportive complementary therapy that can possibly help reduce hot flashes, improve sleep, and ease your anxiety and unpredictable mood symptoms (Johnson et al., 2019; Balzer, 2021; Cefaratti-Bertin, 2023). Acupuncture entails the gentle insertion of thin needles into specific energy-bearing places on your body, aiming to restore balance and promote overall well-being.

Herbs and Dietary Supplements

Herbal and dietary supplements like black cohosh, flaxseed, soy, and vitamin E—to name just a few—are frequently utilized for fighting menopause symptoms (*Menopausal Symptoms: In Depth*, 2017). Nevertheless, more studies are being conducted to ascertain their efficacy. So far, no supplement has unfailingly demonstrated superior usefulness compared to HRT in managing VMS. Keep in mind that these supplements won't grant you superpowers, but they may provide a slight boost. It's always a good idea to talk to your doctor before taking any herbal supplements, especially if you're on other medications, just to make sure everything plays nicely together (WebMD Editorial Contributors, n.d.-d.).

Black cohosh is a cool plant that grows in North America and has been used by Native Americans for a long time (Mohapatra et al., 2022). It's like a superhero for women's health. It's a phytoestrogen that acts like estrogen, and because of this, it's really good at relieving menopause symptoms. It may also benefit you if you suffer from polycystic ovarian syndrome or fibroids. If you drink black cohosh, you may experience side effects like digestive problems, nausea, breast or muscle pain, infections, and problems with sensitive skin. Be careful because it can also affect your health if you have liver problems, and it can interact negatively with certain medications. For example, if you are on hormonal birth control, black cohosh can impact its effectiveness as it changes your hormone levels (Shoemaker, 2024). Black cohosh may be used in combination with other supplements like St. John's wort for menopause (Chung et al., 2007).

Soy and Equol Products

Soy and equol products may help reduce hot flashes. Without complicating things too much, let's talk about the differences between them. Soy, which is rich in daidzein, tends to be the most useful for female health. Daidzein is a substance that can transform into equol within the digestive system. Equol is a substance that mimics some of the effects of estrogen by binding to estrogen receptors in the body (Merz, 2017).

Unfortunately, only about half of Asian women and a quarter of Caucasian women have the required bacteria in their intestines to convert daidzein into equol. As a result, equol supplements might be more useful than soy for some women. Preliminary investigations suggest that taking a 10-mg S-equol supplement twice a day could help manage hot flashes without serious side effects. Nevertheless, further studies are required to be certain that it really helps (Merz, 2017).

Flaxseed

Flaxseed is made up of omega-3 fatty acids, fiber, alpha-linolenic acid, and phytoestrogens named lignans, which are comparable to estrogen. Flaxseed is used to treat obesity as it contains a lot of fiber to curb cravings, and it helps ease constipation and control high blood sugar and hyperlipidemia. It also helps alleviate kidney swelling and rheumatoid arthritis in females diagnosed with autoimmune conditions because of its anti-inflammatory properties (*Flaxseed - Uses, Side Effects, and More*, n.d.).

Here are some other benefits of taking flaxseed for menopausal symptoms (*Flaxseed Oil Benefits & Side Effects*, 2019):

- **Reduces inflammation:** Flaxseed contains alpha-linolenic acid, which has anti-inflammatory properties that may help decrease inflammation and assist with treating bowel-related issues.
- **Stops hair problems in their tracks:** Because of all the nutrients in flaxseed oil, it is used for dry scalp conditions, hair loss, and overall hair wellness. And it will make your nails shiny too!
- **Improves cholesterol levels:** Flaxseed may help lessen total cholesterol or "bad" cholesterol levels.
- **Reduces the chances of getting breast cancer:** Flaxseed contains lignans, which may help decrease your chances of getting breast cancer.

Even though flaxseed is considered safe for the majority of people, some uncomfortable side effects are possible, such as bloating, stomach pain, and diarrhea. If you are diabetic, it's better to steer clear of using flaxseed oil as it will lower your blood sugar too much and put your health in danger. Make sure you stop using it well before planned surgery, as it may raise your chances of bleeding. Flaxseed interacts with many medications, so you need to talk to your doctor before starting to use it if you are on other medications (*Flaxseed Oil Benefits & Side Effects*, 2019; *Flaxseed - Uses, Side Effects, and More*, n.d.).

Dong Quai

Dong quai, also called female ginseng, is an herb that is used in Chinese medicine to help with menopause (*Dong Quai*, n.d.). Some say it can help with specific symptoms like hot flashes, but research isn't clear (Heitz, 2019; *Dong Quai - Uses, Side Effects, and More*, n.d.). Combining it with other products may help with menopause symptoms, but just taking dong quai by itself doesn't seem to do much (Hirata et al., 1997).

Common side effects of taking dong quai include passing gas, high blood pressure, feeling bloated, and an increased sensitivity to sunlight. Consumption of dong quai can also cause skin inflammation and rashes.

Taking dong quai in high doses over a period of six months may not be safe (*Dong Quai - Uses, Side Effects, and More*, n.d.). Dong quai can mimic estrogen and accelerate the progress of certain diseases, so if you have breast cancer, uterine cancer, ovarian cancer, or any other hormone-sensitive condition like endometriosis or uterine fibroids, you should avoid its use. Additionally, it may increase the risk of bleeding and bruising, which can be especially dangerous for individuals with bleeding disorders or those who are undergoing surgery (Ames, 2023). If you want to make good use of this herb, it is best to consult a licensed traditional Chinese medical doctor. They will use a combination of herbal medicines to treat your symptoms holistically (*Dong Quai: Purported Benefits, Side Effects & More*, 2023).

Red Clover

Cows and other animals munch on red clover. Red clover has these natural chemicals called isoflavones, which act like estrogen in our bodies. These isoflavones might help treat menopause-related issues like hot flashes and heart health (*Red Clover*, n.d.-a).

Red clover is also believed to help with conditions like frail and fragile bones, breast pain, and eczema. According to Ehsanpour et al., scientific studies have shown that red clover supplementation can have a desirable effect on the quality of life in post-menopausal women (2012). However, other sources disagree, stating that although red clover is commonly used to treat menopausal symptoms, there is limited evidence to support that it actually works (*Red Clover - Uses, Side Effects, and More*, n.d.). Despite this, red clover continues to be a favored supplement among women seeking alternative ways to manage menopausal symptoms.

Talk to your doctor before using red clover, especially if you have a hormone-sensitive condition as red clover's estrogenic activity may affect you (Davidson, 2020; *Red Clover - Uses, Side Effects,* and More, n.d.).

Evening Primrose Oil

Evening primrose oil is made from the seeds of the *Oenothera biennis* plant. Many people believe that it can help reduce common menopausal issues including hair loss, trouble sleeping, anxiety, and joint aches (*The Benefits of Evening Primrose Oil During Menopause*, n.d.). Some studies indicate that evening primrose oil has shown promise in lessening the intensity and regularity of night sweats in postmenopausal women (Kazemi et al., 2021).

The oil contains an omega-6 fatty acid named gamma-linolenic acid (GLA), which is known for its antioxidant, pain-relieving, and anti-inflammatory properties. GLA has the potential to alleviate symptoms associated with PMS, such as back pain, digestive problems, feeling tired, breast tenderness or pain, feelings of sadness, depression, and grouchiness (WebMD Editorial Contributors, n.d.-a).

Evening primrose oil can be used in two forms: gel (capsules) and oil (bottled). The daily recommended dosage is 500 mg (*The Benefits of Evening Primrose Oil During Menopause*, n.d.). It's important to talk to your doctor before using evening primrose oil, especially if you're taking medications like anticoagulant, antipsychotic, or anticlotting medications that can cause a severe interaction. You might experience some side effects like an upset stomach, headaches, and feeling queasy.

Homeopathic Remedies

Homeopathy is an integrative system of medicine that treats you holistically rather than treating a specific condition or symptom you are experiencing. It has the potential to be beneficial in maintaining your health while going through menopause and addressing various symptoms (Grimley, n.d.). However, the evidence for the efficacy of homeopathy in managing menopause symptoms is limited.

Homeopathy is a form of medicine where the original substance is diluted to the point where it is no longer present. This makes it safe to use without any side effects, and low-potency remedies are readily available. However, for optimal results, it's important to select the right remedy that matches most of your symptoms. Therefore, it is recommended to consult a certified homeopath who will thoroughly assess your symptoms and choose the most suitable remedy for you. A typical consultation usually lasts around an hour to discuss your symptoms, followed by subsequent sessions to review and adjust the remedy's potency as necessary.

Lachesis Muta

Lachesis, extracted from the poison of the bushmaster snake, is thought to alleviate symptoms such as hot flashes and hormonal imbalances. It may specifically address issues like excessive sweating at night, grouchiness, jealousy, headaches, depression, hemorrhages, general weakness, and sleep disturbances (*Know Your Remedy: Lachesis*, n.d.).

Sepia

Sepia—obtained from the cuttlefish's ink bag—is used to help with symptoms related to depression, exhaustion, and hormonal changes, especially during menopause. It can be helpful if you are feeling worthless or depressed, your self-confidence is low, or if you want to isolate yourself as well as if you are uninterested in sex or experiencing discomfort during intercourse. Sepia is often suggested for women who feel tired, irritable, and indifferent toward their loved ones. It can also be beneficial for postnatal depression and hormonal changes during all stages of a female's reproductive life. Sepia may offer relief for vaginal infection, psoriasis, left-sided headaches, fatigue, and feelings of overload and burnout (Herndon, 2021).

Cimicifuga

Cimicifuga, a popular over-the-counter homeopathic remedy made from black cohosh, is thought to be helpful for menopausal symptoms like excessive sweating at night, changes in mood, sudden feelings of heat, a dry vagina, lightheadedness, and feeling down in the dumps. Cimicifuga is also known for its ability to help with irregular periods, headaches, and joint pain (Mohapatra et al., 2022).

Other Homeopathic Remedies

- **Folliculinum:** This is suitable for hormonal symptoms during menopause, especially for women who have used contraceptives or have a history of abuse. It can help with feeling drained and relationship issues (Appleby, n.d.).
- **Sulfuric acid:** This can be helpful if you are experiencing debility or weakness, you're having nightmares, or you feel irritated most of the time (Appleby, n.d.).
- **Graphites:** This can be helpful for improved mood and decision-making, managing your weight, and alleviating constipation during menopause (Sharma, n.d.-a).
- **Adamas:** This can be used for bladder problems linked to women suffering from dry vagina issues. It's made from the dust of diamonds (Worden, n.d.).
- **Ignatia:** This is known for its effectiveness in addressing depression, sadness, and a desire to be left alone during menopause. You may consider trying this if you're suffering from spiraling moods (Sharma, n.d.-a).
- **Phosphorus:** Recommended for women experiencing tooth pains or nose and gum bleeds as well as women with anxiety or who experience joint pain, irregular bleeding, and restlessness (Sharma, n.d.-b).

To find the most suitable remedy for your symptoms, it's important to study different remedies. Choose one remedy that you feel is the best fit. Remember to use only one remedy at a time and

- **Ylang-ylang:** Assists in regulating sebum secretion, minimizing dandruff, diminishing hair breakage, and enhancing hair texture.
- **Rosemary:** Has the ability to promote hair growth by stimulating the growth of hair follicles and increasing their depth. It contributes to overall hair health.
- **Thyme:** This oil helps your hair grow and prevents hair loss. It can also be used to treat conditions like dandruff and hair loss, including conditions like alopecia areata.
- **Lavender:** Known for its calming and relaxing properties, lavender oil is great for promoting hair growth.
- **Cedarwood:** This oil has properties that can fight against fungal and bacterial infections. It can also promote blood circulation and reduce dandruff and has been found to help treat hair loss when combined with lavender and rosemary oils. Additionally, it can be used to treat conditions like alopecia areata.
- **Clary sage:** Clary sage oil can help hair to get stronger and improve your hair growth, making your hair less likely to break.
- **Tea tree:** Tea tree oil has antimicrobial and antibacterial properties and can help treat dandruff and scalp conditions that may contribute to hair loss.
- **Lemongrass:** Lemongrass oil can help clarify the scalp, remove buildup, and promote hair growth.

To use essential oils for hair loss, simply mix a few drops with a carrier oil, such as coconut oil, jojoba oil, or olive oil, and massage it into your scalp. You can also add a few drops to your shampoo or conditioner.

Sexual Dysfunction During Menopause

Essential oils can help manage sexual dysfunction. Lavender and neroli, and combinations of the aforementioned involving geranium, fennel, and rose, may improve your sexual activity (Khadivzadeh et al., 2018).

Take Caution During Use

Returning home after a demanding day at work to the delightful fragrance of your favorite essential oil can instantly alleviate stress. Indulging in a soothing bubble bath infused with a pleasant scent can make you feel rejuvenated. However, essential oils can also be hazardous, potentially leading to chemical burns and even fatalities. The popularity of aromatherapy is on the rise, but it must be approached with caution and proper knowledge to ensure safety. You may want to really study it before use. Here are some important tips to keep in mind when using essential oils (Siegmund-Roach, 2015):

- **Get your oils from a reliable source:** It's really important to purchase your essential oils from a source you can trust. That way, you know they're good quality and pure.
- **Follow instructions and dosages:** Always read and follow the instructions that come with the essential oils. They will tell you how much to use for different purposes. Never consume essential oils orally.
- **Do a skin test first:** Before using a new essential oil, it's a good idea to do a skin patch test. Here's what you need to do: Put a little bit of watered-down oil on your skin and see if anything happens. Oils like oregano and thyme red can make your skin itchy and cause allergic reactions, even if they are diluted because these are really strong oils, so

make sure to dilute those oils even more before you use them.

- **Introduce oils one at a time:** When experimenting with new essential oils, it's advisable to introduce them individually to determine if there are any allergic responses or sensitivities to a specific oil.
- **Take extra care if you have asthma:** If you have asthma or any other health condition, it's important to be cautious when using essential oils. Some oils may trigger asthma symptoms, so it's a good idea to talk to an aromatherapy professional before using them.
- **Keep to expiration dates and follow proper storage guidelines:** Essential oils can become more potent as they age. If you're using essential oils for therapeutic purposes, it's important to store them correctly and avoid using expired oils.

If you experience any irritation, redness, or reaction, stop use immediately. If you follow these rules, you can safely enjoy the benefits of essential oils while reducing the chance of harmful reactions.

Now that we have covered all the nitty-gritty details, let's shift our focus to discussing how you can embrace a nourishing and supportive lifestyle to navigate through menopause with vitality and well-being. The next chapter focuses on the second component of the 7-Component BALANCE Framework: Adopting healthy nutrition.

3

ADOPTING HEALTHY NUTRITION

After her divorce, Jillian's weight drastically increased. Everyday things she used to do and even the hobbies she loved the most were no longer possible. Working in her garden, walking on the beach, cleaning her apartment, or even walking from her car to her office without losing her breath became impossible. And the worst part—she was only 52 years old. How would she feel at 65? Would she even make it that far?

Jillian realized that she needed emotional support to stop the emotional eating spree she was on, but that was not all she needed —she had to change her lifestyle. So she started exercising and, most importantly, she became mindful of her eating habits.

Just like Jillian, we all face our own challenges when it comes to our eating habits, weight, and health. Each of us has unique physical and health-related obstacles to overcome. Fortunately, there are numerous options available to help us transform our lifestyles and adopt healthier eating habits.

FUELING YOUR MENOPAUSAL JOURNEY: NUTRITION ESSENTIALS

I want you to adopt the right mindset. Instead of thinking of a specific diet, welcome the idea of a lifelong lifestyle change—and then do it!

Yes, we will be discussing some specific eating strategies (let's not call them diets, okay?), but first, I want to lay a general framework for what your body needs as a woman in her menopausal years. Thereafter, we'll discuss some specific eating strategies, and through trial and error, you can test and adapt your strategy according to what works for you because everyone's body has its unique needs.

Nutrition in Menopause: A General Framework

Bring the rainbow into your diet and add a little sunshine too. If you want to be well, you need to eat different kinds of foods. Be mindful of your choices by reading labels on food packages to support a healthy lifestyle.

Ensure you get enough calcium by consuming calcium-rich foods daily, such as dairy—preferably yogurt for the good bacteria, which can also help you digest lactose—and fish like sardines and canned salmon along with broccoli, dark leafy vegetables like kale and spinach, and legumes like black beans and peas. Aim for a daily calcium intake of 1,200 mg (Harvard Health Publishing, 2022).

We know calcium is good for our bone health, but vitamin D is also needed for proper absorption. Together, these vitamins fight osteoporosis, so remember to get some sunshine every day or take vitamin D supplements if the weather does not allow for time spent outdoors.

By incorporating a minimum of three servings of iron-rich foods into your daily meal intake, you can boost your iron levels. Some examples of foods high in iron include poultry like chicken and eggs, lean red meat, fish like hake, a variety of nuts, whole or fortified grains like wheat flour, and leafy greens. The suggested daily requirement for iron in older women is 8 mg (WebMD Editorial Contributors, n.d.-c).

Prioritize fiber-rich foods to support your health. Aim for approximately 25 g of fiber per day (Yeager, 2022). To reach this goal, include cereals, rice, whole grain breads, fresh fruits, pasta, and vegetables in your diet.

Achieve and maintain a healthy weight by embracing portion control and enjoying a balanced diet. Remember, skipping meals is a no-no! If you need guidance, reach out to a registered dietitian or consult with your doctor to find your ideal body weight.

Remember, ladies, a colorful plate is a happy plate! Make sure that when you eat, half of your plate is covered in delicious fruit or veggies (*Healthy Eating as You Age*, n.d.).

Slow down on the consumption of high-fat foods. Ensure that fat makes up no more than 35% of your daily calorie intake. Restrict saturated and trans fats (like full-cream dairy and margarine) to less than 7% of your daily intake. These are killers when it comes to raised cholesterol and heart health (WebMD Editorial Contributors, n.d.-c). Add good fats to your diet, such as monounsaturated fats in flaxseed, omega-3 from fish, and olive oil.

Consume sugar and salt in smaller quantities, and when it comes to salt-cured and smoked foods, try to consume and enjoy them on a limited basis. Excessive sodium intake is associated with elevated blood pressure (WebMD Editorial Contributors, n.d.-c). So let's sprinkle just the right amount of salt on our food, like a pinch of stardust. The same applies to sugar; it's the killer of all things good and stands in the way of healing your body, halting your wellness journey.

Avoid highly processed and instant foods as much as possible. They have lower nutritional values and are often full of additives. Remember, freshly cooked food is always better—and it tastes real too!

If possible, don't drink alcohol at all. Restrict your intake to one (or no) drink per occasion, and drink only on special occasions. Instead, stay hydrated by keeping up with the general rule of consuming eight glasses of water each day. This fulfills the daily quota for most fit grown-ups. Imagine sipping on those eight glasses of water like a thirsty marathon runner reaching for the finish line!

THE MEDITERRANEAN DIET

The Mediterranean diet is a plant-centered approach. It promotes eating foods that are packed with important nutrients like fiber, vitamins, and minerals. These include legumes, beans, vegetables, fruits, whole grains, nuts, and seeds. Olive oil is the main source of fat in this diet, while fish and poultry are consumed in moderate amounts, and red meat and processed foods are limited. If you follow this lifestyle, you will include more natural spices and steer away from using salt.

Think of the Mediterranean-style diet as being the cool kid on the block, emphasizing the consumption of good carbs and fats.

Saturated fat, trans fat, and cholesterol are the bad guys here. But fear not—we have some heroes too: monounsaturated fats (i.e., nuts and olive oil) and polyunsaturated fats (i.e., fish oils and flaxseed). The Mediterranean diet knows how to strike the perfect balance with a moderate amount of fat, mostly coming from these healthful fats and unsaturated omega-3 fats. It's like a superhero squad for your taste buds!

The Mediterranean diet has various health advantages, including better gut health, increased longevity, improved brain health, and a lower risk for certain cancers, type 2 diabetes, and cardiovascular disease (Davis et al., 2015). Not only is the Mediterranean diet healthy, but it is also tasty and easy to follow, making it a popular choice if you're looking to enhance your overall health and well-being.

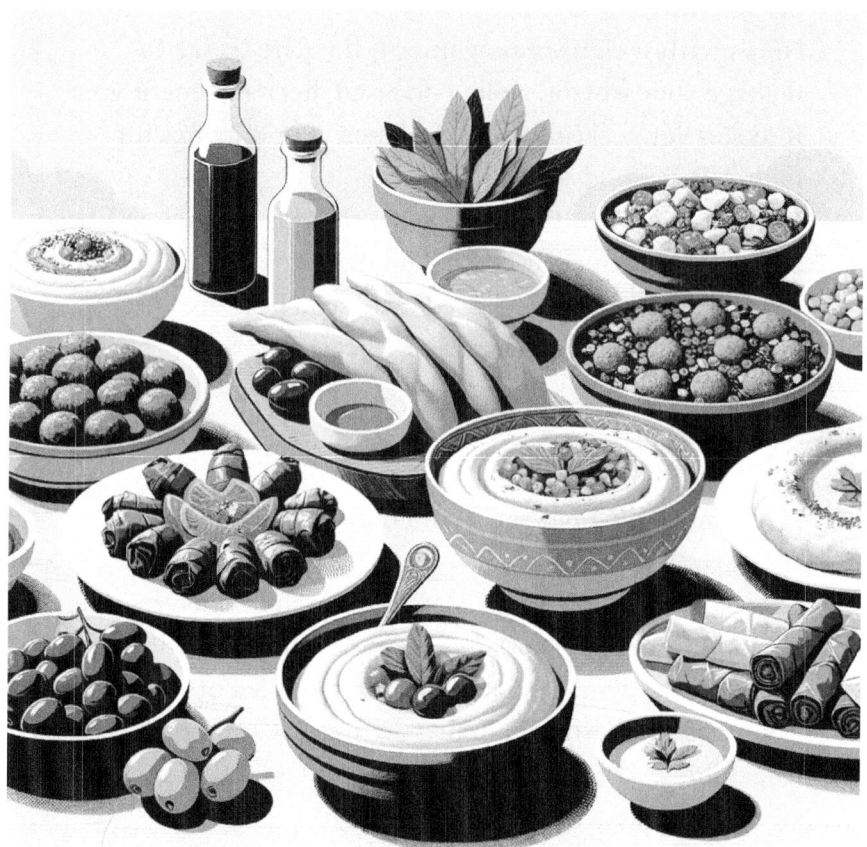

Plant-Focused Foods

A diet consisting of plants? Yup, it's all about eating lots of different vegetables, fruits, whole grains, legumes, beans, nuts, and seeds. Here are some of the main advantages of this lifestyle:

- **Lots of nutrients:** These foods are loaded with vitamins, minerals, fiber, and antioxidants that are great for your health, especially fresh fruits and vegetables.
- **Lower risk of chronic diseases:** Eating lots of fruits and veggies has been linked to reducing the prevalence of diabetes and certain cancers and a lower risk of heart disease (Kubala, 2023b).
- **Helps with weight management:** If you're trying to manage your weight, a plant-focused diet can benefit you. It makes you feel full and can reduce your cravings for high-calorie foods.
- **Improves gut health:** Plant-focused foods are high in fiber and great for your gut health and digestion.
- **Cost-effective:** Plant-focused meals can be more cost-effective than meals that include meat.

Fiber-Rich Portions

Here are some high-fiber foods and their fiber content:

- **Fruits:** Pears, apples, and berries are high in fiber, making them some of the fiber superheroes of the fruit world! For example, the average pear provides about 5 g of fiber, giving your digestive system a high-five (Gunnars, 2023)!
- **Vegetables:** Artichokes and broccoli are good sources of fiber. For instance, one cup of these little green trees

provides around 2 g of fiber. Plus, they're delicious too (Gunnars, 2023)!

- **Grains:** Fiber-rich foods such as oats, barley, brown rice, and whole wheat are excellent sources of whole grains. One cup of cooked barley contains about 6 g of fiber, which is enough to keep your digestive system happy and your taste buds entertained (*31 High-Fiber Foods You Should Be Eating*, 2023)!
- **Legumes:** Kidney beans, peas, and baked beans are high in fiber. Lentils are a good source of fiber too. For instance, one cup of cooked lentils provides nearly 16 g of fiber (O'Brien, 2023). So go ahead and enjoy these fiber-packed delights!

Healthy Fats

Healthy fats from olive oil, nuts, seeds, and avocados offer various benefits for heart health and cholesterol reduction. Nuts and seeds are great providers of unsaturated fats, which help bring down low-density lipoprotein (LDL) cholesterol that is not good for your health. By lowering your LDL, your body maintains stable blood pressure and healthy blood vessels (*Nuts and Seeds*, n.d.). Olive oil is abundant in beneficial monounsaturated fats and antioxidants, which have the potential to diminish the likelihood of heart disease, decrease blood pressure, and alleviate inflammation (Leech, 2023). Plus, these delicious ingredients add a sprinkle of heart-healthy goodness to your meals! Additionally, seeds contain healthy monounsaturated and polyunsaturated fats, which can help reduce inflammation and cholesterol levels, contributing to better heart health.

Moderate Dairy Products

Low-fat dairy items, like cheese and yogurt, should be included in intermediate quantities in your dietary habits. Low-fat dairy products contain essential nutrients like calcium, B vitamins, protein, and vitamin D (*Dairy*, n.d.). Nevertheless, it is crucial to exercise caution when consuming dairy products that have a high fat content as they may contain saturated fats. These fats have been connected with an elevated risk of heart disease. According to the 2015–2020 Dietary Guidelines for Americans, it is suggested that adults and children over nine years old should have three 1-cup (8 oz) servings of no-fat or low-fat milk, yogurt, or other dairy foods each day. This helps promote calcium intake and lowers the risk of certain diseases (*2015–2020 Dietary Guidelines*, n.d.). So while enjoying moderate amounts of low-fat dairy products can promote better bone health and provide essential nutrients, it's important to choose low or no-fat options to limit saturated fat intake.

If you prefer a vegan or nondairy diet, there are numerous dairy substitutes to consider. Options like almonds, cashews, oats, or soy milk are not only rich in calcium but also contain other essential nutrients.

Poultry and Fish

Consuming fatty fish like salmon and mackerel on a regular basis is advised as part of a healthy diet. These types of fish are abundant in omega-3 fatty acids, which have been proven to have anti-inflammatory attributes, help lessen blood pressure, and bring down the likelihood of heart disease (Giosuè et al., 2022). Poultry is a great protein provider and can be part of a healthy diet in limited quantities. Select only lean cuts of poultry and avoid eating the skin as it contains high levels of saturated fat (Davis et al., 2015). The Mediterranean diet, which includes regularly eating fatty fish, has been connected with various health benefits, including better brain health and a lower prevalence of heart disease (Lordan et al., 2018).

Manage Your Red Meat Intake

The limited intake of red meat is a key aspect of the Mediterranean diet, which focuses on plant-focused foods and offers various health benefits.

Here are some tips to follow when it comes to eating red meat (*Limit Red and Processed Meat*, n.d.):

- **Limit your red meat intake:** A maximum of three portions of red meat per week is recommended. The size of three portions shouldn't exceed 500 g (18 oz).
- **Choose lean cuts:** When you do eat red meat, opt for leaner cuts. This helps you consume lower amounts of saturated fat.
- **Try poultry and fish:** If you're looking for alternatives to red meat, fish or poultry are great options.
- **Include legumes and beans:** Instead of relying solely on red meat, consider incorporating legumes, beans, and lentils into your diet. They offer essential nutrients and fiber.
- **Remember other sources of nutrients:** While red meat does provide important nutrients like iron, protein, vitamin B12, and zinc, you can also find these nutrients in other foods like poultry, fish, and plant-focused options.

Red meat should be your side dish as opposed to your main course. Keep it limited to avoid increased risk of cancer, diabetes, heart disease, and even early death (Harvard Health Publishing, 2020a). Plant-focused protein options cost less and provide you with the same benefits as red meat, such as supplementing your zinc levels.

If the thought of going meatless for an entire day doesn't tickle your taste buds, why not start with a few meatless meals every week? You have the flexibility to organize your schedule based on your preferred meatless meals, like pasta, vegetable lasagna, salad, and yummy soups like butternut or broccoli. Alternatively, you can experiment by swapping out meat for some protein-rich alternatives in your go-to recipes. For instance, you can add lentils and beans to salads, stews, and soups. If you're craving burritos or tacos, try using refried vegetarian beans. And if you're into stir-fry dishes, toss in some tofu for a delicious twist (Mayo Clinic Staff, 2022b)!

Herbs and Spicy Food

Herbs and spices are really important for making food taste better, and they can help reduce the need for using too much salt. This is good for keeping your blood pressure in a healthy range and promoting heart-healthy dietary habits (Institute of Medicine, 2010). While we don't know as much about the health benefits of herbs and spices compared to salt, they might have the potential to lower blood pressure. A recent study discovered that increasing the inclusion of herbs and spices in meals resulted in lower readings in blood pressure over 24 hours (Lambert, 2021).

In addition, simply using spices and herbs instead of salt can make a great difference. Think of processed foods; these already contain a high sodium content. Adding more salt to already salty food can be very dangerous for your health. It makes more sense to replace it with some herbs or spices. What I mean is that spices and herbs can actually help us meet the suggested amount of sodium in our diet. It's really important to watch how much sodium we eat because it helps lower blood pressure and reduces the risk of heart problems (Silva-Santos et al., 2022).

Including different herbs and spices in your cooking can be a helpful way for women who want to control their blood pressure and improve their heart health. But remember what we discussed earlier: If you are struggling with night sweats or angry hot flashes, it's best to manage your spicy food intake because you're hot enough already!

Don't Wine Too Much

The Mediterranean diet sometimes includes drinking a moderate amount of wine, especially red wine, with meals (Davis et al., 2015). People believe this is good for your health. Red wine has antioxidants like resveratrol, which might reduce your blood pressure and lower cholesterol and, as a result, protect your heart from an attack. But it's important to know that drinking too much alcohol can be bad for you. It can make you gain some weight, cause liver disease, and increase your chances of developing certain cancers and some serious heart problems. So while people on the Mediterranean diet may enjoy a moderate amount of wine, it's important to follow the recommended guidelines for alcohol and be aware of the risks of drinking too much. Cheers to a balanced lifestyle!

Other Things to Consider

The Mediterranean diet is not only about what you eat. Being active, sharing the same lifestyle with the people close to you, and creating a relaxed and social atmosphere during meals are necessary too. These things are deeply rooted in the traditional Mediterranean lifestyle. Maintaining a healthy weight, developing better eating habits, and improving overall health have been linked to eating meals together as a family.

Staying frequently active outdoors is also a big part of the Mediterranean lifestyle, which helps promote wellness and good health. The Mediterranean diet also highlights the value of enjoying meals with others and taking time to relax after eating, like by taking a siesta. Your wellness and overall health can experience positive effects from these practices.

The Benefits of Following a Mediterranean Lifestyle

Try the Mediterranean diet, a healthy way of eating that can help women going through menopause feel better and find solace from symptoms. Indulge in whole foods, from vibrant fruits and veggies to wholesome grains, seeds, nuts, beans, and olive oil (Durward, 2022).

By following this diet, your inflammation will become less—yup, hopefully you'll experience less joint pain and stomach discomfort—and you will feel a decrease in the common menopausal symptoms you are experiencing, like hot flashes, night sweats, and depression. As an added bonus, it also helps with reducing pesky belly fat and weight control as obesity is a big problem for many women during menopause (Dweck, 2022). Foods like vegetables, fruits, and olive oil have great anti-inflammatory benefits.

The Mediterranean diet is loaded with nutrients from seasonal fruit and vegetables, which can further help minimize menopausal symptoms and support overall health (Roach, n.d.). We've already covered the benefits of a plant-focused diet, but just to recap, it includes lots of nutrients, lowers the risk of chronic diseases, helps with weight management, improves gut health, and is cost-effective.

Did you know that women going through menopause have a higher chance of developing heart disease? Don't worry, there's a delicious solution! The Mediterranean diet is packed with heart-healthy fats from nuts and fish. These fats can actually improve your heart health and keep your cholesterol levels in check, reducing the risk of heart disease.

Oh, and let's not forget about bone health! During menopause, it's common for bone density to decrease, which can be a bit concerning. But guess what? The Mediterranean diet has got your back on that too! It's loaded with calcium and vitamin D from dairy products, fish, and leafy greens. These nutrients can support your bone health and help counteract the effects of decreased bone density during menopause.

I understand different cultures have different diet and food preferences, so it's okay if you choose and adapt some aspects of this diet to fit your own needs and preferences. But if you think there is nothing to lose, why not give the Mediterranean diet a try? It's not only good for your heart but also your bones. Here's to a healthier you!

SUPPLEMENTS THAT WORK WELL

Although following a healthy diet like the Mediterranean diet will help you get your required daily nutrients, you may need some extra help if you can't include all those nutrients in your diet for whatever reason. The good news is that there are some supplements that are worth a try.

There are several supplements that can support women during menopause, but it's important to consult with a doctor before taking any supplements to make sure they're safe and suitable for your specific needs.

Multivitamin Supplements

According to Hillary Wright, a registered dietitian, the top-rated all-around supplement for menopause is Bayer's One A Day Women's Menopause Multivitamin (Younkin, 2023). This supplement includes essential nutrients such as magnesium, vitamin D, and calcium to promote healthy bones. It also contains zinc and biotin, which may aid in reducing hair loss. Moreover, this multivitamin includes naturally occurring compounds found in soybeans called soy isoflavones that provide estrogen-like effects to your body.

It's also filled with the isoflavones genistein, glycitein, and daidzein, which have been demonstrated to alleviate night sweats and hot flashes (Younkin, 2023). A study revealed that women in early menopause with a six-month intake of soy protein with isoflavones are prone to fewer cardiovascular risks (Sathyapalan et al., 2018).

Even if you can't find Bayer's One A Day Women's Menopause Multivitamin where you live, you may be able to compare the ingredients on alternatives to find a similar product with multivitamin components as there are many different products available for menopause support.

In Chapter 2, we talked about other alternative medicines that may help alleviate menopausal symptoms, including black cohosh, flaxseed, and red clover. Now, let's take a look at which vitamins may assist you specifically. Vitamins A, D, E, B6, and B12 are all essential vitamins that can support you during menopause (McDermott, 2023).

Specific Vitamin Support

- **Vitamin A:** During menopause, low estrogen levels can be mitigated with a set of retinoids found in vitamin A, which supports your bone health, vision, and immune function and can be found in foods such as leafy greens, carrots, and sweet potatoes. Avoid overdosage as too much vitamin A may lead to negative effects. Taking high doses of vitamin A for a long time can cause dizziness, nausea, headaches, and, in severe cases, liver damage. Pregnant women should be careful not to take excessive amounts of vitamin A as it can increase the risk of birth defects. While vitamin A is important for bone health, excessive intake can weaken bones and increase the risk of fractures. When it comes to managing bone health and decreasing your risk for fractures, it is better to avoid consuming high doses of vitamin A, which is typically present in animal-sourced products like eggs, liver, and fish as well as supplements and fortified foods. Instead, it is suggested that women consume moderate dosages of vitamin A sourced from beta-carotene, which is derived from vegetables and fruit (Harvard Health Publishing, 2014). Additionally, high doses of preformed vitamin A can cause skin changes like dryness, itching, and increased sensitivity to sunlight. Opting for plant-focused sources of vitamin A and sticking to the suggested intake amounts is a safer option (Kubala, 2023a).

- **Vitamin B6:** This B vitamin is important for brain function and the production of neurotransmitters such as serotonin and dopamine. It can help alleviate symptoms such as mood swings and depression during menopause. Foods like avocados, salmon, chickpeas, and bananas are rich sources of Vitamin B6. Taking too much vitamin B6 can have negative effects on your body, such as having difficulty focusing, feeling irritated or anxious, experiencing depression, experiencing short-term memory loss, and having muscle weakness. Taking very high doses of vitamin B6, specifically 200 mg or more per day, can lead to neurological disorders such as balance issues and loss of feeling in your legs. In rare cases, allergic skin reactions have been reported in response to high doses of vitamin B6 supplements. Other possible side effects include bleeding easily if you're on blood thinning medication, sensitivity to sunlight, headaches, nausea, abdominal pain, and loss of appetite (McDermott, 2023; *Vitamin B6*, n.d.).

- **Vitamin B12:** This vitamin provides great support for nerve function and blood cell production as well as alleviating symptoms such as mood swings and fatigue during menopause. Vitamin B12 is present in animal-derived foods like fish, meat, and dairy and in some yeast and fortified cereals. Consuming excessive amounts of vitamin B12 can have negative effects, such as feelings of facial swelling, nausea, sweating, irregular heartbeat, fatigue, an increase in weight, vomiting, diarrhea, and others. Although rare, some individuals have reported allergic skin reactions when taking high doses of vitamin B12 supplements. Vitamin B12 can interact with certain medications such as antibiotics and antihypertensive medications used for high blood pressure (McDermott, 2023; *Vitamin B12 Deficiency*, n.d.; *Vitamin B12 Side Effects*, n.d.).

- **Vitamin D:** Vitamin D is important for bone health and immune function. It can help alleviate symptoms such as joint pain and muscle weakness during menopause. Vitamin D can be found in fatty fish, egg yolks, and fortified products such as milk and breakfast cereal (WebMD Editorial Contributors, n.d.-f). However, it can be challenging to get enough vitamin D from food alone, so taking supplements is a good idea. Exercise caution as excessive intake of vitamin D can result in various side effects, such as queasiness, vomiting, reduced appetite, weakness, weight loss, constipation, confusion, heart rhythm issues, kidney stones, and kidney damage. In severe cases, excessive vitamin D intake can lead to changes in mental health and kidney problems (Spritzler & Kubala, 2024).

- **Vitamin E:** Do you bruise easily? Are you constantly struggling with dry skin or thinning hair? Feeling like a walking polka dot with age spots on your skin? Experiencing a libido that's taken an unexpected vacation? Battling memory and concentration problems that make you feel like a scatterbrained detective? Catching colds and viruses faster than a superhero catches villains? And let's not forget those pesky leg cramps that make you dance the crampy tango! Well, it might just be time to check your vitamin E levels! Vitamin E is a versatile nutrient that offers multiple benefits. It helps reduce menopausal symptoms and manage anxiety (Feduniw et al., 2022). As a powerful antioxidant, vitamin E supports your journey through menopause by fighting free radicals that damage your cells by reducing inflammation (*Let's Get to the Facts*, n.d.). Not only does vitamin E act as a superhero for your heart by preventing clotting and protecting against age-related diseases, but it also boosts your immune system and helps ward off infections. You can find vitamin E in foods like seeds, nuts, vegetable oils, and avocado. The daily intake is suggested at 15 mg. That's roughly like enjoying 2 tbsp of peanut butter, munching on two dozen almonds, or savoring a creamy avocado (Crowther, n.d.). So why not give those hot flashes a run for their money with a daily dose of vitamin E? Remember to follow the recommended guidelines for a happy and healthy experience with vitamin E! Too much vitamin E may lead to side effects such as stomach pain, diarrhea, exhaustion, headaches, queasiness, itchy rashes, blurred eyesight, and feeling frail. Also, 400 units or more per day can have negative effects on your body, including an increased chance of having a stroke or heart problems and even death. Vitamin E can also interact negatively with other medications and supplements. If you have bleeding disorders, are vitamin K-deficient, have diabetes, or have a history of heart or liver disease, it is best to avoid high doses (American Heart Association, 2004; Mayo Clinic Staff, 2023d).

WHY WEIGHT LOSS IS HARD DURING MENOPAUSE

When menopause comes knocking on your door, you'll experience quite a lot of hormonal changes and a decrease in muscle mass, which ultimately makes weight loss more challenging. Are you gaining weight rapidly and don't know why? Some things that can cause your weight to increase during this time are lower estrogen levels, losing muscle as you get older, lifestyle choices like what you eat and how much you exercise, and symptoms of menopause like feeling down, experiencing hot flashes, and having trouble sleeping (*Menopause and Weight*, n.d.).

Tips to Lose Weight

Being a woman is a blessing, but it's not without a curse or two. Managing body weight is definitely on that list for many of us. Despite the challenges that come with menopause, it's important to prioritize a healthy lifestyle to manage your weight. Here are some easy ways you can do so (*Menopause and Weight*, n.d.):

- **Stay active:** Regular exercise can aid in weight loss and maintaining a healthy weight.
- **Eat well:** Focus on a balanced diet that includes whole, unprocessed foods. Minimize your intake of highly processed foods and added sugars. This will support your hormonal health as well as your weight loss goals.
- **Limit alcohol:** Cutting back on alcohol can contribute to better weight management and overall well-being.
- **Get enough sleep:** Adequate sleep is crucial for your overall health and hormonal balance. Every night, try to get at least 7–8 hours of proper sleep.
- **Manage your stress:** Chronic stress can affect your appetite-regulating hormones, leading to increased calorie intake and weight gain. Use restorative practices to handle stress, such as partaking in activities you love and following mindfulness techniques (Harvard Health Publishing, 2021).

If you can include these strategies in your daily routine, you will be better able to maintain a healthy weight and support your wellness during menopause.

Talk to your doctor about your weight and possible hormone replacement therapy as this may help to control your weight too.

How to Control Your Weight to Keep It Stable

Stick to Weight-Control Basics

- **Diet:** Maintain a balanced eating plan that incorporates a diverse range of fruits, vegetables, whole grains, lean sources of protein, and nourishing fats. Be mindful of portion control to manage calorie intake effectively.
- **Physical activity:** Regular exercise is important for weight management. Include a mix of aerobic exercises, such as brisk walking, swimming, or cycling, and strength training to enhance your metabolism and muscle mass.
- **Stress management:** Use stress-reducing activities like meditation, deep breathing exercises, yoga, or hobbies to help prevent yourself from emotional eating and for your overall emotional and physical wellness.

Eat a Balanced Diet

- **Nutrient-rich foods:** Eating nutrient-dense foods will help you meet your increased nutritional needs during menopause. Consume calcium-rich foods for bone health and foods rich in fiber to support your digestion.
- **Hydration:** Remember to stay well-hydrated as proper hydration is essential for the proper function of your metabolism and your overall health.

Exercise Regularly

- **Aerobic exercise:** A minimum of 150 minutes of moderate-intensity aerobic exercise is suggested weekly (Yang, 2019). Activities like swimming, dancing, and brisk walking can be enjoyable and beneficial.
- **Strength training:** At least twice a week, incorporate strength training exercises to keep your muscle mass intact as it tends to decline during menopause (*Why Exercising After Menopause Is Important*, n.d.). This can also help counteract the natural decrease in metabolism. We'll talk more about staying active in Chapter 4.

Prioritize Sleep

- **Sleep hygiene:** Practice better sleep habits by maintaining a consistent sleep schedule and creating a comfortable sleep environment. Remember to limit your caffeine intake after midday.

Manage Stress

- **Stress-reducing techniques:** Use techniques to manage your stress, such as mindfulness, meditation, progressive muscle relaxation, and engaging in activities you love. Stress reduction can positively impact both mental and physical health.

Consider Hormone Therapy Cautiously

- **Consult with your doctor:** You need to talk to your doctor before considering hormone therapy during menopause.

- **Individualized approach:** Pursuing hormone therapy should be individualized, considering factors such as medical history, personal preferences, and potential risks and benefits.
- **Quality over quantity:** Both the duration and quality of your sleep are important. Poor sleep can disrupt hormonal balance and contribute to weight gain.

While you are going through menopause, it's really important to understand how nutrition affects your weight. By following a balanced diet that includes healthy foods packed with nutrients and staying active with regular exercise, you can overcome the difficulties of gaining weight during menopause. This will help you achieve your desired weight and overall health goals.

With the right knowledge and dedication, menopause can become a positive phase where you regain control of your body and embrace a healthy and energetic lifestyle. Investing in physical activity and nutrition is valuable for your body's well-being. That's what we are going to talk about in the next chapter.

4

LIVING ACTIVELY

This chapter dives into the third component of the 7-Component BALANCE Framework: (L): Living actively. Chapter 4 will take you on a journey through the exciting world of exercise during menopause, covering everything from safety precautions to a wide range of workouts. Get ready to explore mind-body practices like yoga and Tai Chi and discover motivation and obstacle-conquering strategies for a healthier, more active life!

EXERCISE? HERE'S WHY!

When it comes to menopause and exercise, I need to share Jane's story. She was a keen exerciser and had a more active lifestyle than most of the women I know, but her menopause experience was the worst—her symptoms combined with her emotional well-being at that stage following the COVID-19 lockdown left her bedbound and unable to exercise. With the encouragement of her friends and fellow gym enthusiasts, and with the help of hormone replacement therapy, she regained the ability to engage in regular exercise. This not only supported her overall health and well-being, but it also allowed her to feel like her true self once more.

Exercise is like Jane's best friend, and it can be for other women experiencing menopause too! It's like a secret weapon that helps keep your muscles strong and your bones healthy all while reducing the chances of any unexpected falls. Plus, it does wonders for your posture, making you stand tall and proud! Not only that, but exercise also brings a sense of calm, flexibility, and balance to your life.

If you're feeling overwhelmed by your symptoms and emotions, why not take a quick 15-minute walk? And if you happen to run into someone you know, it's even better! A quick chat or a smile can truly make a world of difference to your day. You've got this! Keep moving and grooving!

Regular physical activity during menopause offers you a multitude of benefits for your physical and mental well-being. In the next section, we'll talk about the key benefits of physical activity during menopause as well as the recommended amount and types of physical activity.

Benefits of Physical Activity During Menopause

- **Improved physical and mental health:** Engaging in regular physical activity can do wonders for your physical health by helping you manage your weight, lowering the risk of chronic diseases, and boosting your overall well-being. And guess what? It's not just your body that benefits! Regular exercise also works its magic on your mental health, reducing the risk of anxiety and depression (Payne, 2021). So let's get moving and feel amazing inside and out!

- **Bettering your vasomotor symptoms:** You know what's great? Regular exercise! It can totally help reduce the intensity and frequency of your menopausal symptoms like hot flashes and night sweats. Studies have shown that physically active women experience milder vasomotor symptoms compared to those who have a less active lifestyle (Kim et al., 2014).
- **Empowering and coping:** Physical activity can give women a boost in dealing with the changes during menopause. It's like having a secret weapon that brings a sense of control and confidence, making this life transition a breeze!

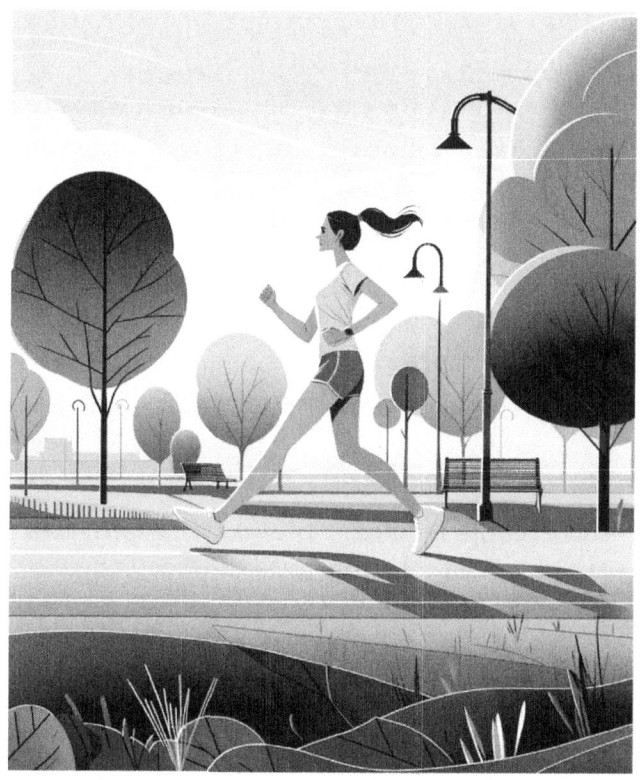

RECOMMENDED AMOUNT AND TYPES OF PHYSICAL ACTIVITY DURING MENOPAUSE

Here's a fun tip for postmenopausal women: Spice up your exercise routine with a delightful blend of aerobic, strength, flexibility, and balance exercises! Check out these general guidelines for staying active during menopause:

- **Aerobic exercise:** Aim for at least 150 minutes of moderate-intensity aerobic exercise per week, and let's get those endorphins dancing (Yang, 2019)!
- **Strength training:** To keep your muscles strong and your bones healthy, make sure to do strength training exercises at least twice a week (*Why Exercising After Menopause Is Important*, n.d.).
- **Flexibility and balance exercises:** Women who are not physically active are more likely to experience mental health problems, and it was found that mild regular exercises in older postmenopausal women benefited them more than an extremely active lifestyle (Felipe et al., 2020). Add exercises like yoga and Tai Chi that help improve flexibility and balance and go for regular walks in between.

EXERCISE AND MENOPAUSE 101

To keep you feeling fabulous, the exercise program for postmenopausal women should include a mix of endurance exercises (aerobic), strength exercises, and balance exercises (Payne, 2021). Aim to squeeze in two or more sessions per week for a total of about two and a half hours and let your inner fitness queen shine! Consider this while exercising:

- **Safety measures:** Before starting any exercise program, it's always a good idea to have a chat with your doctor, especially if you have any existing medical conditions. They'll help ensure you're on the right track to a healthier you!
- **Aerobic exercises:** Rev up your cardiovascular system and have a blast with moderate-intensity aerobic exercise each week. Think brisk walking, swimming, or cycling—the choice is yours!
- **Strength training:** To keep your muscles strong and your bones healthy, make sure to include strength training exercises in your routine at least twice a week. It's like giving your body a little extra oomph! However, if you have chronic issues with bone health, make sure you don't engage in high-intensity exercises that may lead to falling (Mishra et al., 2011).
- **Balancing exercises:** Improve your posture and reduce the risk of falls with some fun balance exercises like yoga! Let's add a little stability and a whole lot of smiles to your fitness routine!
- **Mind-body practices:** Yoga and Tai Chi promote relaxation, flexibility, and balance. Let's get our Zen on and find our inner balance!
- **Stress management:** Take a chill without a pill and try stress-reducing techniques like meditation, deep breathing exercises, or progressive muscle relaxation to keep your cool and boost your overall well-being!
- **Hydration:** Stay well-hydrated before, during, and after exercise to maintain energy levels and prevent muscle cramps—because nobody wants to feel like a dried-up raisin!

- **Get some quality sleep:** Prioritize quality sleep. Remember, a good night's rest not only helps you feel refreshed but also keeps those pesky hormones in check, preventing unwanted weight gain!

MINDFUL MOVEMENT

Yoga for Menopausal Women: A Fun and Refreshing Approach!

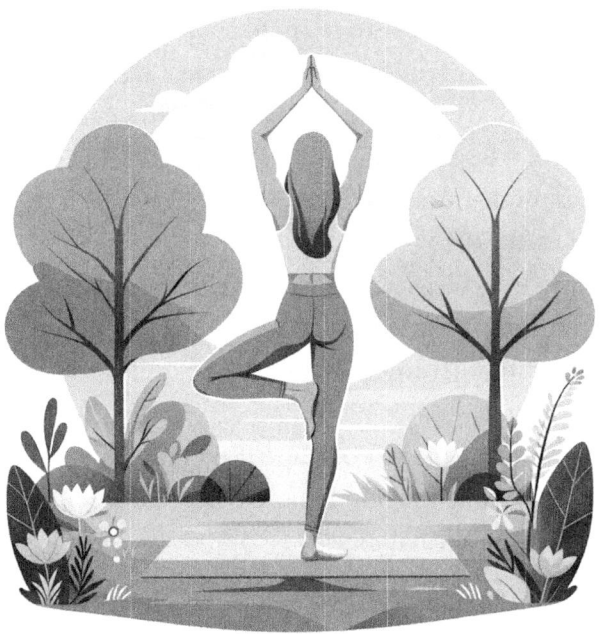

Yoga can help you manage the physical and psychological symptoms of menopause. It involves specially adapted yoga poses, breathing techniques, and mindful meditation exercises to support you during this stage of life (Coveney, 2013). So strike a pose, find your inner Zen, and let those hot flashes flow away like a gentle breeze!

Some of the benefits of yoga for managing menopause symptoms include (Coveney, 2013):

- **Manage stress and better your sleep:** Yoga can help relieve stress, anxiety, and insomnia associated with menopause.
- **Relieving the effects of menopause:** Yoga has been shown to significantly reduce overall symptoms of menopause, such as muscle and joint pain, hot flashes, and night sweats.
- **Boosting physical strength:** Yoga can help maintain bone density, muscle strength, and balance, which can help prevent falls and other injuries.
- **Improving mental resilience:** Yoga helps realign your emotions, such as mood swings, anxiety, and depression.
- **Supporting positive thoughts:** Yoga can help to support positive thinking that boosts your self-worth.
- **Recharging drained energy:** Yoga can help you manage hot flashes, alleviate joint and muscle pains, and recharge drained energy caused by insomnia and fatigue.

Yoga is an amazing practice that brings a whole range of benefits to menopausal women. Let's start with some gentle warm-up exercises like neck rolls and shoulder rolls to get those muscles nice and loose. It's like giving your body a friendly wake-up call before diving into the practice. And hey, don't forget about the deep breathing exercises during the warm-up! They work wonders in calming the mind and reducing stress, which is super important for managing those pesky menopausal symptoms.

Now, let's dive into some specific yoga recommendations tailored just for you.

Hot Flashes and Night Sweats? No Problem!

We've got some cooling poses up our sleeves, like forward folds, seated forward bends, and supported bridge poses. These poses are like a refreshing breeze that can help alleviate those hot flashes and night sweats. Ahh, sweet relief!

Anxiety and Depression? We've Got Your Back!

Try out some poses that are all about relaxation and grounding, such as the child's pose, the legs-up-the-wall pose, or even the peaceful corpse pose. These poses are like a warm hug for your mind, helping you manage anxiety and depression with ease.

Bone Density and Balance? We've Got You Covered!

Let's get those bones strong and steady with some weight-bearing poses. Strike a pose in tree pose, warrior pose, or even the challenging chair pose. These poses are like a secret weapon for maintaining bone density and improving balance. You'll feel like a superhero!

Need Some Rest and Rejuvenation? We've Got Just the Thing!

Time to unwind and recharge with some restorative poses. Imagine yourself in supported fish pose, supported reclining bound angle pose, or simply kicking your legs up the wall. These poses are like a mini vacation for your body, helping you relax and rejuvenate.

Zen Your Way to Bliss: Unwind and Meditate!

Finish off your practice with a blissful relaxation or meditation session. It's like the cherry on top, promoting overall well-being and leaving you feeling refreshed and centered.

If you are a yoga newbie, you can find information on all these poses on the Yoga Journal website by using their Pose Finder feature. So grab your yoga mat and let's move toward a fitter you!

Tai Chi for Menopausal Women

Tai Chi, with its gentle flowing movements, is another excellent option for menopausal women.

When you practice Tai Chi, you engage in an exercise that combines meditation, movement, and breathing, and it has a low impact on your body. It has been found to offer numerous benefits for women going through menopause, and several studies have discovered that practicing Tai Chi can help reduce the frequency and severity of hot flashes and night sweats in menopausal women. Additionally, Tai Chi has been found to enhance the quality of sleep, which can alleviate fatigue and other symptoms experienced during menopause (*Tai Chi for Menopause Symptoms*, n.d.).

By practicing Tai Chi, you are engaging in a form of meditation that aids in reducing stress and anxiety, which are common symptoms of menopause. Moreover, Tai Chi has been associated with various overall health benefits, including enhanced mental well-being, improved cardiovascular health, and increased flexibility and muscle strength.

In fact, one study suggests that Tai Chi could be one of the most effective exercises for targeting and alleviating menopausal symptoms. It can help reduce insulin resistance and related physiological risk factors for cardiovascular disease, improve your mood, well-being, and sleep, reduce your chance of getting comorbidities like diabetes, enhance your bone health, and help you manage your weight effectively (*Tai Chi for Menopause Symptoms*, n.d.; Whiteley, n.d.). Here's how to start:

- **Gentle warm-up:** Begin with a gentle warm-up, including stretching and joint rotations, to ease into your Tai Chi practice.
- **Deep breathing techniques:** Practice deep breathing techniques to relax your body and mind before diving into the movements.
- **Basic Tai Chi movements:** Start with basic Tai Chi movements like the Tai Chi stance, shifting weight, and flowing movements. It's like dancing with tranquility!
- **Balance, flexibility, and strength:** Focus on movements that promote balance, flexibility, and strength, such as "Grasp the Sparrow's Tail" and "Wave Hands Like Clouds." Feel the grace and power in each motion!
- **Mindfulness and meditation:** Incorporate mindfulness and meditation into your Tai Chi practice to enhance the mind-body connection and find your inner Zen.
- **Gradual progression:** As you become more comfortable and experienced, gradually increase the intensity and complexity of your Tai Chi practice. It's a journey of growth and self-discovery!

If this is the first time you're trying out Tai Chi, don't be scared! There are many online sources, including videos on YouTube, to help you out. Websites like Tai Chi Basics and CureJoy give clear instructions on how to do the basic moves.

SAMPLE EXERCISE PLAN

Your journey to achieving strong bones, increased strength, and a fabulous body composition relies heavily on your sleep habits and nutrition (Atkinson, 2020). Don't underestimate the power of these factors! If you don't provide your body with enough calories and protein, you won't have the necessary ingredients for muscle growth. But fear not! The loss of muscle that comes with aging is not a permanent sentence. It can be avoided and even reversed!

When it comes to protein, make sure you're getting it from high-quality sources, especially around your strength training and high-intensity interval workouts. This is the perfect time for your body to use protein and make the most of your efforts (Atkinson, 2020). And remember, rest is just as important as exercise, so be sure to prioritize proper rest, and that includes getting enough sleep. Your body will thank you!

A sample exercise program for menopausal women should include a combination of aerobic, strength training, and flexibility exercises. The below program does not reflect Saturdays and Sundays, as these are your rest days, but if you want to swap the days around, you are welcome to compile your own personalized program (Atkinson, 2020):

Week	Monday	Tuesday	Wednesday	Thursday	Friday
1 & 2	Strength training: 1set of 20 repetitions	Low to moderate exercise: Brisk walking for 20 minutes	Low to moderate exercise: Yoga for 15 minutes	Low to moderate exercise: Brisk walking for 20 minutes	Strength training: 1 set of 20 repetitions
3 & 4	Strength training: 1 set of 20 repetitions	Low to moderate exercise: Brisk walking for 25 minutes	10 minutes of interval training Low to moderate exercise: Yoga for 15 minutes	Low to moderate exercise: Brisk walking for 25 minutes	Strength training: 1 set of 20 repetitions
5 & 6	Strength training: 2 sets of 20 repetitions	10 minutes of interval training Low to moderate exercise: Yoga for 15 minutes	Low to moderate exercise: Brisk walking for 30 minutes	Strength training: 2 sets of 20 repetitions	Low to moderate exercise: Brisk walking for 30 minutes
7 & 8	Strength training: 3 sets of 20 repetitions	Low to moderate exercise: Brisk walking for 30 minutes	15 minutes of interval training Low to moderate exercise: Yoga for 20 minutes	Strength training: 3 sets of 20 repetitions	15 minutes of interval training Low to moderate exercise: Yoga for 20 minutes

Make sure to warm up before starting your routine and remember to cool down as soon as you're finished. Be sure to add some brief stretching exercises into your daily routine to help improve flexibility, prevent injuries, and enhance your overall mobility.

Strength Training

On the days you have strength training, make sure you pick a minimum of four to a maximum of six upper-body exercises and a minimum of two to a maximum of four lower-body exercises. You are welcome to do any activities of your choice, but here are some suggestions:

- **Upper-body strength:** Bicep curls, shoulder raises, and chest presses.
- **Lower-body strength:** Wall sits, leg deadlifts one at a time, squats, and lunges.

Websites like MuscleWiki.com and BodyBuilding.com are great resources for learning how to do different types of activities and which muscle groups each activity targets.

Interval Training

Interval training is a type of workout where you do a series of exercises for different lengths of time. The work interval is where you work really hard for a specific distance or amount of time, and the recovery interval follows when you take it easy for a little while. You can change how fast you go, how long you exercise, and how much rest you take to reach different fitness goals during your training session (Goulding, 2022).

Activities like swimming, rowing, running, and cycling are perfect choices for interval training. They allow you to challenge yourself more than you would in a nonstop workout. You can basically pick any activity or exercise that you like to do as long as you remember to put in all of your effort so that you end up out of breath and totally exhausted. For example, if you're planning to do intervals for 10 minutes, you can jog fast for 3 minutes, walk for 30 seconds, jog fast again for another 3 minutes, and walk again for 30 seconds, continuing this until your 10 minutes are done.

Low to Moderate Exercise

These types of activities include things like swimming, brisk walking, dancing with slow steps, jogging, lifting light weights, practicing Pilates, or leisurely riding your bicycle.

This workout example is solely provided for informational purposes. It's really important to talk to a professional before starting a new exercise program, especially if you have any health concerns or haven't exercised for a long time. They can provide personalized guidance based on your specific needs. If possible, exercise under the supervision of a qualified trainer to ensure proper form and technique.

Now that we've exercised your body, let's exercise your mind and heart. In the upcoming chapter, we'll talk about practices that nurture mental and emotional well-being and delve into techniques for resilience, stress management, and finding inner peace. Through mindfulness exercises, relaxation techniques, and insights into emotional strength, you will discover tools to navigate life's challenges with grace and fortitude to reinforce the interconnectedness of mind and body in the journey toward optimal health.

Before we move on….

"The miracle is this: The more we share the more we have."

— LEONARD NIMOY

Hey there, superhero!

Menopause is like a roller coaster for your body and mind. But guess what? We've got *The Ultimate Guide to Menopause* to help you master this wild ride with confidence and ease. This book is your trusty companion to make your menopausal journey a breeze. What do you think about sharing this knowledge and making a difference?

Why should you share your thoughts on this book? Well, think of it this way: You are not just leaving a review; you are extending a helping hand to someone out there who is in the same boat you once were. They are looking for answers, guidance, and a friend to help make menopause less of a mystery.

Wouldn't you want to be that friendly face who guides them through it all?

Our mission is simple—make menopause knowledge accessible to everyone. Everything we do revolves around that mission. And to achieve it, we need your voice. Yes, yours!

Many people judge a book by its reviews, and your words can be the beacon of light for someone trying to navigate the choppy waters of menopause.

So here's the deal: Will you lend a hand to fellow women by leaving a review for this book? Your gift takes less than 60 seconds but can change another woman's life forever.

Your review could help...

...another woman embraces the journey of menopause.
...one more good friend trying to support her bestie through the changes.
...a busy mother understands and celebrates this natural transition.
....one more person to achieve holistic wellness and confidence.

To make a real difference, all you have to do is scan the QR code below with your phone camera and leave your review on Amazon.com:

If you purchased the book from another Amazon site, you can go to "Your Orders" in your account, choose the book, and click "Write a product review".

If you're up for being a superhero for someone you've never met, you're in the right place. Welcome to the club! You're now one of us.

I'm beyond excited to share valuable insights that will make your menopausal journey smoother and more enjoyable. Get ready to discover the secrets within the upcoming chapters.

Thank you from the depths of my heart. Now, let's get back to making this menopausal journey an adventure worth celebrating!

Your biggest fan,

Hera Bennett

PS - Did you know that sharing something valuable makes you more valuable to others? If you think this book will help another friend on their menopausal journey, pass it on. Sharing is caring!

5

ACHIEVING INNER PEACE AND RESILIENCE

I n this chapter, we'll talk about the fourth component of the 7-Component BALANCE Framework: (A): Achieving inner peace and resilience. Chapter 5 explores the profound mind-body connection and techniques to bolster mental and emotional well-being. It emphasizes the practice of meditation and mindfulness for cultivating your inner harmony and resilience. So let's get into it!

FINDING THE RIGHT SUPPORT ON YOUR JOURNEY

Janet has faced a roller coaster of challenges due to hormone-related and gynecological issues that have impacted her life, career, and relationships. Picture this: dealing with intense premenstrual syndrome and heavy periods at just 16, a diagnosis of endometriosis, many heartbreaking miscarriages, the stress of fertility treatments, managing pregnancy, motherhood, and postnatal depression, and, to add the cherry on top, grappling with menopausal symptoms. It's been a tough journey, to say the least.

Through it all, she sought help, tried different treatments, and faced some discouraging reactions. The turning point came when a gynecologist actually listened, believed her, and reassured her that she wasn't grappling with a mental illness. That was the game-changer. It led to the discovery of a hormonal imbalance, a result of having her ovaries removed, and finally getting the right hormonal replacement. And guess what? It made a world of difference to her well-being.

Janet's story shows us the importance of being heard and understood when you're dealing with health challenges. It's about finding the right support and treatment. Her journey highlights how crucial it is to recognize and address hormonal imbalances, especially with conditions like endometriosis, fertility issues, and menopause. It also throws light on the real-life consequences of misdiagnosis and the need for healthcare providers to pay attention to and believe patients' experiences. I guess what I want to say is if your doctor does not believe you, support you, or try to find a solution to your symptoms, you need to find one who is willing to walk the crazy and confusing path of menopause with you.

Here's the uplifting part of Janet's story—her resilience shines through, and she experienced positive outcomes after finally getting the right care. They're not just a win for her; they're a beacon of inspiration for anyone else out there wrestling with similar struggles. The right help and understanding can truly make a life-changing difference.

Take Better Care of Yourself

All those physical changes during menopause can affect your self-esteem and confidence, and it's important to give yourself time and space to adapt to these changes.

Take time for self-care activities like having a cup of tea, reading a book, going for a walk, or practicing mindful breathing exercises. Make sure you connect with other women experiencing menopause so you can support each other and have people to talk to who understand what you're going through. Find an online support group or create a personal group among your friends. You need to know that you have to prioritize caring for yourself. You simply cannot help and support others if you don't help yourself first. Fill your cup, and then serve from it.

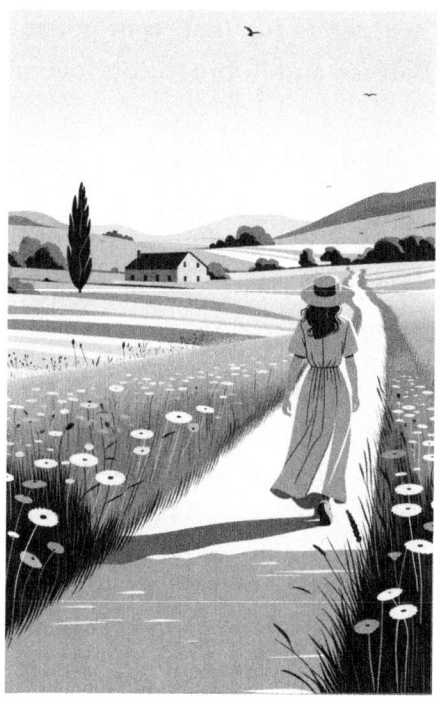

YOUR MIND-BODY CONNECTION

Let's talk about something super important: the mind-body connection. A scientific connection! It's basically understanding how our thoughts and feelings can team up with our physical health. It's like realizing that your mood and emotions can throw a party in your body without your permission (*What Is the Mind-Body Connection?*, 2019).

Let's break it down: Chronic stress and the blues can team up to bring on health issues like cardiovascular health problems, a weakened immune system, and digestive drama. You need to be emotionally resilient to face these physical challenges head-on.

Positive vibes, a tough-as-nails mindset, and some solid coping strategies can be lifesavers for your physical health and well-being. The mind-body connection isn't just about getting in touch with your feelings; it's a reminder that your mental and emotional health is like the Batman and Robin to your overall body health.

Benefits of a Great Mind-Body Connection

Here's the deal: stress and negativity? They're like the bad guys, weakening your immune system and making you more likely to get sick. Nobody wants that, right?

Now, the good news: Mindfulness, meditation, yoga, and CBT can be like superheroes. They combat inflammation, enhance your immune system, and contribute to an overall improvement in your well-being. It's akin to treating your body to a mini spa retreat!

And guess what? The mind-body connection isn't just about health —it's your emotional "best friend forever" too. Ever tried yoga? It's like a chill pill, helping you relax, reducing anxiety, and lifting your mood. We all need that sometimes, especially during menopause.

A great mind-body connection is all about deciding daily what's right for you. It's like having the power to decide what's best for your body and mind. You're in control!

So let's get real. By understanding and taking care of this mind-body thing, you're giving yourself the VIP treatment. Teaming up your brain with your body is your greatest strategy to keep your menopause symptoms at bay! Think mindfulness, meditation, and a few tricks from cognitive behavioral therapy. They're not just fancy words; they're your secret weapons for feeling awesome emotionally and rocking it physically. It's like a double win for your well-being during this menopausal journey! You've got this!

MENOPAUSE AND MENTAL WELL-BEING

During menopause, a lot of women encounter stress, depression, and anxiety. Menopausal symptoms that are commonly experienced can include various things, such as feeling easily irritated or angry, having a decrease in self-esteem and confidence, feeling down, having trouble concentrating and being forgetful—sometimes called "brain fog"—and struggling to find the right words (*Menopause and Your Mental Wellbeing*, 2022). But hey, at least you'll always have an excuse for forgetting things!

Your symptoms can be worsened by problems with sleep and tiredness. It is important to seek help and support if you are struggling with mental symptoms during menopause. Treatment options include cognitive behavioral therapy (CBT), hormone replacement therapy (HRT), counseling, and mindfulness. Exercising regularly and eating a balanced, nutritious diet can help improve your menopausal symptoms (*Menopause and Your Heart*, n.d.). Now you know why we've covered all these topics in previous chapters.

Here are some of the key mental health aspects affected during menopause (Harvard Health Publishing, 2020b):

- **Mood changes:** For women who have a history of mental health issues, menopause can lead to even worse mood swings, irritability, and anxiety, often attributed to fluctuating hormone levels, particularly decreasing estrogen.

- **Depression:** Menopause can bring about an elevated likelihood of encountering significant episodes of depression, and it is not uncommon for certain women to endure depression for the first time in their lives.
- **Anxiety:** Menopause can also be associated with an increased risk of anxiety, including the potential for panic attacks during and after this transition.
- **Difficulty sleeping:** Night sweats and hot flashes, common symptoms of menopause, can contribute to sleep problems, which in turn can impact mood and overall mental well-being. Difficulty falling asleep or staying asleep will make you tired all day long and affect your mood.
- **Impacting current mental health issues:** Menopause can worsen existing mental health conditions like schizophrenia and bipolar mood disorder (*How Menopause Affects Your Mental Health*, n.d.). It's important for women and their healthcare providers to be aware of these potential impacts and to address them proactively.

The influence of decreasing estrogen levels during menopause is a key factor in these mental health changes. Estrogen has been shown to have a modulating effect on mood, and its decline during menopause can contribute to the onset or exacerbation of these mental health symptoms.

MENOPAUSE AND EMOTIONAL WELL-BEING

Did you know that negative thoughts can drain your energy? Your thoughts have the power to shape your physical and emotional health. Choose thoughts that uplift and empower you!

Menopause and emotional well-being are like "besties" or "worsties," depending on how you manage them. Your hormones during this period can take your emotions on a wild ride. You need to be aware of these emotional changes and take steps to maintain your emotional well-being.

Mood swings, irritability, and anxiety—the menopausal transition can be a time of psychological difficulties, and it's essential for women to be aware of these potential emotional impacts.

During menopause, the way you feel emotionally can be affected by things like changes in your hormones, stress, and what's going on in your personal life (Holland, 2020). Once you feel conflict pouring over you like a heat wave, take a deep breath and think it over before you react impulsively. Don't allow menopause to ruin your relationships. Manage your emotions before they manage you.

Taking care of your emotional well-being is just as important as managing physical symptoms during menopause. This may involve practicing stress reduction techniques, engaging in regular physical activity, and maintaining a healthy diet. It's essential to find time for yourself during the day, even if it's just for a brief period of relaxation or mindfulness exercises.

How to Manage Your Stress

By gaining a deeper understanding of the impact of menopause on emotional well-being and proactively taking steps to maintain good mental health, women can navigate this transitional period of their lives with more ease and confidence.

Take care of yourself during menopause by incorporating these simple practices into your daily routine (Davis, n.d.):

- **Build your tribe:** Positive and supportive people—that's who you need around you. Whether it's joining a community group, book club, or crafting circle, solid friendships help you feel connected and supported.
- **Don't worry about what you can't control:** Focusing on the things you have the power to influence can help you maintain confidence and a positive mindset.
- **Stand up for yourself respectfully:** Calmly and confidently speak up for yourself without resorting to angry or aggressive forms of communication.
- **Stay active:** Regular exercise not only improves your overall health but also reduces stress, enhances your mood, and benefits your sleep habits.
- **Take time to relax:** Find activities that help you feel centered and relaxed. Things like calming music, relaxation apps, self-care, yoga, and meditation can help you find the calm within the storm.
- **Look on the bright side:** Remind yourself of all the good things in your life and take time to practice gratitude.
- **Find new hobbies and passions:** Have you ever wanted to try something but didn't feel confident enough to do so? Now is the time to take risks and try something new. You may find a hidden talent or even make new friends.
- **Prioritize rest:** Ensuring you get enough good-quality sleep is essential to keep your mind and body functioning optimally.
- **Journal:** Jotting down your thoughts and feelings can be a helpful way to reduce stress. If you prefer other creative outlets, you can try coloring, drawing, diamond-dotting, or painting.

- **Eat well:** Eating a well-rounded and healthy diet can help your mental health and stress levels as well. Avoid alcohol and reduce your caffeine intake, perhaps grabbing a soothing herbal tea to take a break instead.

MORE ABOUT MINDFULNESS, MEDITATION, AND RELAXATION

In Chapter 2, we dipped our toes into the world of meditation and mindfulness. Why? Because they're like secret weapons against stress, sleep struggles, and the ups and downs of menopause. Let's face it, menopause is "me(a)n" and it often feels like there is "no pause." Think of meditation and mindfulness as your personal helpers for feeling awesome again.

But here's the cool part: These practices aren't just about relaxation. Nope, they're like a crash course in understanding yourself better and understanding how to get emotional balance in your life. Picture it as having a superpower that comes in handy during this wild ride of life changes. So let's keep this in mind: Meditation and mindfulness are your go-to buddies for not just surviving but thriving through menopause.

How Body Scan Meditation Works

Body scan meditation is a mindfulness exercise that focuses on directing awareness to the sensations experienced in various areas of the body. It is a valuable technique for promoting relaxation, reducing stress, and increasing self-awareness. Here's some practical information on body scan meditation (Scott, 2021):

- **Find a comfortable position:** Get cozy by finding a comfortable spot, whether it's lying down or sitting up straight with good posture. Take a few deep breaths to center your mind.
- **Begin the scan:** Begin by closing your eyes and directing your attention to your breath. Next, choose a starting point, either the top of your head or the soles of your feet, and systematically move your focus to each area of your body in turn.
- **Notice sensations:** When you're focusing on each body part, be mindful of any sensations you're experiencing, like tingling, tightness, or discomfort. The aim is to observe and acknowledge these sensations without passing judgment.
- **Release tension:** If you're dealing with any tension or discomfort, try to let go of that tension as you exhale and keep taking deep breaths. It might help you feel better!
- **Complete the scan:** Ensure that you complete the scan thoroughly, drawing attention to every part of your body, whether starting from your head and moving down or starting from your toes and moving up.
- **Stop the practice:** Take a few deep breaths and slowly open your eyes when you are ready to finish. Reflect on how you feel before resuming your regular activities.

Benefits of Body Scan Meditation

- **Stress reduction:** Body scan meditation can help reduce stress and promote relaxation by increasing awareness of bodily sensations and releasing physical tension.
- **Improved self-awareness:** This practice can help individuals become more aware of their feelings and

emotions, promoting a greater understanding of their body and mind.

- **Enhanced mindfulness:** By focusing on each part of the body, individuals can develop a deeper sense of mindfulness and presence, which can be beneficial for overall well-being.

Menopause is a transitional phase, but it can last a long time, so taking care of yourself both physically and emotionally can make a significant difference in your well-being. You're not alone, and with these practices, you can navigate this journey.

Guided Meditations in Menopause

Guided meditation is a helpful tool for managing symptoms and improving emotional well-being. Beginners or people who like step-by-step guidance in their meditation practice can find these resources really helpful. Here are some key points to understand about guided meditations for menopause:

- Many guided meditations are available online that offer a natural menopause treatment through imagery and affirmations to provide relaxation and relief from those pesky symptoms.
- When used as a coping strategy for menopause, guided meditations can contribute to empowerment, self-confidence, and an improved sense of control over life and the processes of change. They can also be effective in enhancing your emotional, social, and financial quality of life (Yazdkhasti et al., 2015).
- Many mindfulness apps offer guided meditations tailored to women experiencing menopause. These apps can

provide structured guidance for individuals who are new to meditation or prefer a more guided approach. Some of these apps include features such as learning to meditate, guided meditations, and music for relaxation. Apps like Insight Timer are popular meditation apps that offer guided meditation to help ease the symptoms of menopause. Find out more on their website at InsightTimer.com.

The objective during mindful moments is not to completely clear your mind but rather to become a spectator of the mind's activity while being compassionate toward yourself. The next step involves creating a pause by taking a deep breath and nonjudgmentally observing your thoughts, emotions, and surroundings. This practice of calmness can effectively reduce stress and help you sleep better, and it can ultimately help you achieve inner balance, health, and new energy (Sood et al., 2019).

Other Ways to Calm Your Inner Crazy

Brace yourself because life has taken a wild turn, and no, it's not just your imagination. We're in the midst of a chaotic tornado where taking care of our parents, raising kids, and working like crazy are all crashing into each other. Gone are the days of blissful ignorance before the internet, cell phones, emails, and the never-ending demand of being available to your friends, family, and colleagues 24/7. Remember when a cup of tea could quickly fix all your frazzled nerves? Ah, those were the days! When the roller coaster ride of menopause throws your mental well-being for a loop—hang in there!

I sometimes joke with my friends that I need a glass of wine at the end of the day. Many of my female friends would respond that they need a glass of wine at the end of every day. But we have it wrong. You see, even if red wine may have its health benefits, too much of anything may not be that great after all.

The moment you start drinking regularly, you may start struggling more with your sleeping routine, being more tired, and feeling like you need to have a drink all over again. Plus, you then drink multiple cups of coffee and add some sugar to get you through the day because you are just too damn tired to keep your eyes open. It doesn't make sense though, does it?

But how do you deal with feeling overwhelmed, burnt out, and tired all the time if your daily wine is not the answer? A better way to approach it is to have a specialist who focuses on menopause run a test to check your hormone levels. Balancing your hormones is an important first step toward feeling better. Many women discover that hormone therapy, as recommended by their specialist, is sufficient to improve their overall well-being. If there is a need for additional evaluation by a psychiatrist who may prescribe antidepressants, these medications tend to work better once your hormonal levels are closer to normal, particularly estrogen.

It may not calm all your storms, but take a nice warm bath and try to relax after a long day. Block time out in your busy schedule to meet with "you." And hey, remember to keep a positive outlook!

As we navigate the complex emotions and physical changes that accompany this phase in our lives, it is crucial to embrace self-care, mindfulness, and self-compassion. In the next chapter, we will talk about how to take care of ourselves and find inner strength to succeed in all areas of life. Let's start this next chapter with open hearts and a strong commitment to unlocking our true potential.

6

NURTURING EMPOWERMENT

In this chapter, we will talk about the fifth part of the BALANCE Framework: (N): Nurturing empowerment. Chapter 6 is all about helping you feel more empowered and confident during menopause. It will give you useful tips and techniques to empower yourself and support other women going through menopause. You'll also find helpful resources and info about support groups to guide you on your journey toward personal empowerment.

JOANNE'S STORY OF EMPOWERMENT

Joanne, a 45-year-old educator, found herself facing unexplained symptoms that disrupted her daily life.

The Beginning of the Change

In her early 40s, Joanne began to observe the initial signs of menopause, which included mood changes and hot flashes. Initially, she attributed these symptoms to the natural process of aging, but as they became more frequent and intense, she realized that menopause might be the cause.

The Struggle With Symptoms

As her menopause progressed, Joanne's symptoms became more persistent and severe. She dealt with debilitating hot flashes, sleep disturbances, and mood swings that affected her work and personal life. It wasn't until she consulted her doctor that she received a proper diagnosis and started exploring treatment options.

Finding Relief and Support

Joanne discovered that making simple lifestyle changes, like adopting a healthy diet, exercising regularly, and practicing stress-reduction techniques such as meditation and yoga, could help alleviate her menopause symptoms. She also found comfort in connecting with support groups and online forums where she could share her experiences with other women going through menopause. This really empowered Joanne to reach out to other women.

Advocating for Change

Through her own experiences, Joanne realized the importance of raising awareness about menopause and providing support for women facing similar challenges. She became an advocate for women's health issues in her community and played a key role in starting a local support group for women experiencing menopause. She also shared her story on various platforms, hoping to inspire and empower other women going through "the change."

A Newfound Sense of Purpose

Joanne's journey through menopause not only taught her valuable lessons about her own health but also inspired her to help others. She found a new sense of purpose in advocating for women's health and supporting them as they navigated the challenges of menopause. Through her work, she has shown that it is possible to find relief and support during this often challenging time in a woman's life.

SELF-EMPOWERMENT: EMBRACE YOUR POWER AND REDEFINE YOUR JOURNEY

Your life may be full of menopause jams, but with the right empowerment strategy, you'll confidently find your way around them. It's really easy to feel overwhelmed by the numerous negative perceptions surrounding menopause and the challenges it brings physically, mentally, and emotionally. However, although you can't control whether you go through menopause or not, you can control how you respond to it.

Experiencing a sense of helplessness can make you feel negative and despondent. There are always choices you can make to regain control no matter what personal challenges you encounter. Embracing this concept is the key to personal empowerment, also known as self-empowerment (Mind Tools Content Team, n.d.).

The moment you decide to equip yourself with the right tools and adopt a growth mindset, you gain the ability to transform menopause into a good experience. This transformation isn't limited to your mental outlook; you can also enhance your physical and emotional well-being during menopause through education, taking action, and prioritizing self-care.

Empowering Your Body

Regular exercise is important for managing weight, keeping hormones balanced, and improving muscle tone. When going through menopause, different types of exercise can help improve your overall fitness, including resistance training, walking, yoga, Pilates, and Tai Chi. But exercise is not all you can do to empower your body. Here are some ideas you can try (*9 Ways to Empower Yourself*, n.d.):

- **Maintain a balanced diet:** It's not that much of a stretch to say that you are what you eat. What you put into your body significantly affects your health—mentally and physically. Menopause symptoms can get worse when you eat sugary or processed foods or drink alcohol. Avoiding alcohol and opting for a diet that includes fruit, nuts, vegetables, legumes, and fish helps your body efficiently absorb and utilize essential vitamins and minerals. A balanced diet helps keep your hormones in check.
- **Find ways to feel beautiful:** The changes in appearance that women experience during menopause can impact our self-esteem. You may experience new complexion problems, and your skin may become less firm and drier. Maintaining a skincare routine is one way to counteract some effects of menopause, and you may even explore using a prescription face cream that targets hormonal issues, giving your self-esteem a healthy boost.
- **Appreciate your body:** Many women of any age feel unhappy with their body or physical appearance, and women experiencing menopause are no different. This dissatisfaction can negatively impact your self-esteem, but try to remember that menopause is a natural phase of life and your body isn't conspiring against you. Remind

yourself that your body can do amazing things and allows you to engage with the world and experience life. Trust that your body will guide you through this stage and do what you can to support it!

- **Indulge in self-care:** Allocate a slice of your day to indulge in self-care activities that promote your well-being, ranging from taking relaxing baths to enjoying a coffee break or pursuing hobbies.

Empowering Your Mind

There are two key aspects to consider when it comes to mental empowerment during menopause. First, it's crucial to prioritize your mental well-being as anxiety, brain fog, and depression are common symptoms experienced during perimenopause and menopause. Second, it's important to educate yourself about this stage in your life. By gaining knowledge, you will be better equipped to make informed decisions regarding your health moving forward. Let's take a look at some ways you can practice self-empowerment (*9 Ways to Empower Yourself*, n.d.):

- **Education is key:** It's important to learn about the signs of menopause and treatments for menopausal symptoms. Even though people are talking more about menopause these days, there are still some things that people don't like to talk about, and many people don't know much about the treatments available. By listening to podcasts, reading self-help guides, subscribing to blogs, and watching videos from trusted sources, you can become more informed about the symptoms of menopause. Having conversations with your doctor and friends or family who have experienced menopause can provide valuable insights on how to navigate through it.

- **Reduce your stress:** You need to take steps to reduce your stress levels in order to maintain good mental and physical well-being. Headaches, irregular sleep patterns, and gastrointestinal problems are some of the physical issues you may experience when you are undergoing profound or long-term stress in your life. Stress has a significant impact on cortisol levels in your body, and when cortisol levels are high, other hormones don't function optimally, which can worsen menopausal symptoms.
- **Get help from a professional:** Whether you are feeling low or experiencing cognitive difficulties, a mental health expert can provide valuable guidance to help you navigate through this difficult phase. Do not allow the negative perception associated with therapy to discourage you from seeking the necessary support to maintain your mental well-being.

During menopause, it may seem like you are not in the driver's seat when it comes to your health, but that's far from the truth. Every positive step you take toward your physical well-being, no matter how small, can make a difference. Choose to be consistent —if you decide to make a change, commit to it to experience the rewards.

SUPPORTING OTHER WOMEN ON THEIR MENOPAUSAL JOURNEY

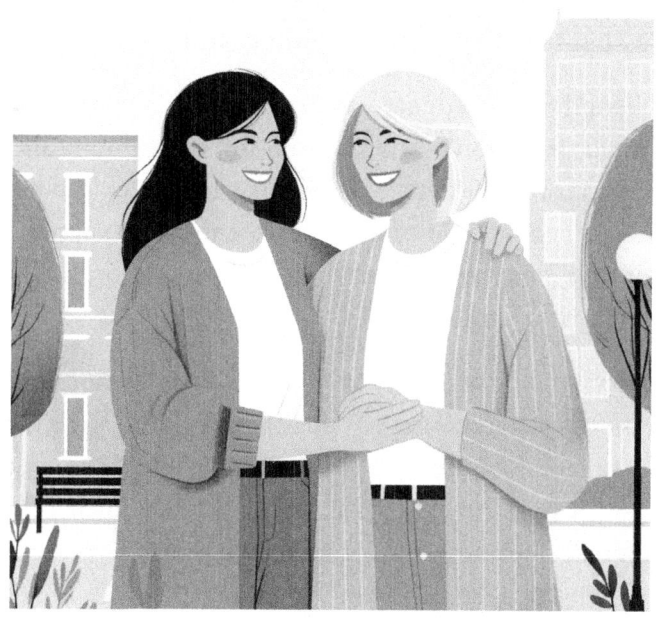

You deserve to have friends who clap loudly when you achieve something, and so do other women. Let's face it: The reality is, at our age, many women don't have many friends or even a best friend anymore. Life happens and people grow apart, move, or even pass away. The fact is that you don't want to face menopause all alone. But the good news is that you don't have to! There are so many other women on the same journey. You just need to find and encourage them. I bet they could use a friend too!

Whether it's an old or a new friend, supporting them through their menopause can be a wonderful opportunity to show them love and care.

Create a warm, welcoming space for them to share their experiences and feelings. Encourage them to make small lifestyle adjustments like staying active, eating well, and avoiding alcohol and smoking. These simple changes can help alleviate menopause symptoms and boost their mood. Lend a helping hand with daily tasks, remind them of their amazing qualities, and offer emotional support by being patient, understanding, and sympathetic.

It's also beneficial to educate yourself about menopause and its physical and emotional symptoms so that you can provide informed support to others. Suggest that they seek guidance from a doctor and consider joining some menopause support groups. Share helpful resources like self-help guides and online forums to foster a sense of community.

Organizations such as Daisy Network, Queer Menopause, The Menopause Charity, Women's Health Concern, and Menopause Matters are great sources of support for those going through menopause. A nice surprise is waiting at the end of this chapter where you will find more resources for support.

Don't forget that each woman's menopause journey is unique, so it's important to avoid assumptions and embrace their personal experience with understanding and support. Believe it or not, most women are not high-maintenance. They don't want tons of advice—they only want a listening ear and to know a friend is near.

HERE'S ONE FOR YOUR SPOUSE OR PARTNER (YUP, HAND THE BOOK OVER...)

If you're reading this, it means your wife or partner is dealing with menopause, and she purchased this book to get the information and support she needs. But I know you'd also like to support her and help her with whatever you can during this time of ups and downs she is facing.

Supporting your spouse or partner through menopause is a journey that requires understanding, empathy, and patience. It's important that you create a safe and open space for them to express their experiences and emotions.

Encouraging healthy lifestyle habits like a balanced diet, regular exercise, and avoiding alcohol and smoking can greatly alleviate symptoms.

Let me share this story with you about a couple I know, let's call them John and Kate. They were happily married with friends and family commenting throughout the years about how in love they were. However, there came a time in their marriage when Kate started complaining of intercourse being painful. John didn't want to hurt her and he started feeling really self-conscious about it, so he stopped pursuing her for physical intimacy. Kate, on the other hand, felt that John's loving and caring approach must have changed all of a sudden because she was no longer attractive to him and did not meet his needs anymore. She was convinced in her mind that John was having an affair. They started arguing a lot and drifted further apart. In the end, they divorced. However, John never stopped loving Kate. After unintentionally listening to an awareness talk on the radio while stuck in traffic, John realized what menopause was and the problems it caused. He also learned that there was help out there for these problems. This made him realize for the first time that if the communication between himself and Kate had been better, if they had both opened up about their true problems and emotions, they could have resolved the problem while it was still small, and perhaps they would have still been happily married. Why am I sharing this with you?

As women go through menopause, hormonal changes in their bodies can often lead to a range of emotional and physical symptoms. One common symptom is increased irritability or mood swings. It's important to understand that these changes are a natural part of the menopausal journey and are not indicative of your wife's true character or personality. The fluctuating levels of hormones can affect neurotransmitters in the brain, which can result in heightened emotions and irritability.

You need to approach these moments with empathy and compassion, recognizing that your partner may be experiencing a wide range of emotions that are beyond her control. Providing support, actively listening, and being patient can go a long way in helping your wife navigate through this challenging phase of her life. Additionally, encouraging her to explore stress-relief techniques, engage in regular exercise, and maintain a healthy lifestyle can contribute to a more balanced emotional well-being. Remember, menopause is a temporary phase, and with understanding and support, both of you can navigate through it together.

Seeking professional help is always an option if needed, and maintaining open communication will strengthen your relationship during this transition. Remind her of her brilliance and the reasons you are together, and reflect on the challenges you have overcome as a team.

Providing practical assistance with daily tasks, such as getting her a refreshing drink or a cool damp towel or even changing the sheets if she wakes up from night sweats, can make a world of difference. Your support and care mean everything to her. In the next chapter, I will also talk about cultivating relationships and how your wife or partner needs to approach their relationships amid all the moods and inner turbulence they are experiencing. You are welcome to join in reading that section too.

BONUS MATERIAL: RESOURCES AND SUPPORT GROUPS

Menopause is a significant life stage that comes with its unique challenges, but you're not alone. Numerous resources and support groups offer information, community, and a helping hand. Let's look at some of the available resources:

Organizations and Websites

North American Menopause Society (NAMS)

Website: www.menopause.org

- Provides information on menopause and related health issues.
- Includes a listing of healthcare providers specializing in menopause.

Hormone Health Network

Website: admin.hormone.org

- Educational resources on menopause, including webinars, podcasts, and fact sheets.

Healthtalk

Website: healthtalk.org

- Provides a platform for women to share their menopausal experiences through videos, audio clips, and written accounts.

- Information on support groups and networks for menopausal women.

Online Support Groups

Peanut Network online community

Website: www.peanut-app.io

- A space for women to connect, share experiences, and ask questions.

Menopause Goddess blog

Website: www.menopausegoddessblog.com

- A blog providing valuable insights and support for women during menopause.

Menopause Matters

Website: www.menopausematters.co.uk

- Provides information and advice on menopause.

Red Hot Mamas

Website: redhotmamas.org

- The biggest menopause learning program in America. You can subscribe to their free online community.

Social Media Support

Menopause support groups on Facebook (Meta)

- **Menopause Support Group:** A large community for sharing experiences and seeking advice.
- **Menopause Solutions by Gennev:** Gennev's Menopause Solutions is a private community overseen by a team of women who specialize in evidence-based menopause care. This inclusive space offers the ideal opportunity to inquire, offer guidance, exchange stories, and acquire knowledge, all while enjoying a good laugh.

Menopause Support on Instagram

- **The Menopause Movement:** Information and tips for managing symptoms.
- **Menopause Support UK:** Provides advice on symptoms and finding healthcare providers.

Mobile Apps

Caria

- Take control of your journey with this empowering user-friendly app for iOS devices designed to support you every step of the way.
- Allows users to track symptoms, access menopause-friendly recipes, and connect with others.

Health & Her

- If you are looking for symptom-tracking tools, guided exercises, and a menstrual cycle monitor, you may want to check out this mobile app for iOS and Android.
- Provides a platform for women to connect and share experiences.

Perry

- A menopause app for iOS and Android with a discussion hub and question-and-answer forum.
- Connects women to share experiences and seek advice.

Navigating menopause can be tough, but with these resources and support groups, you can access valuable information, emotional support, and a sense of community. You're not alone in this journey. Explore these options and find what works best for you—because support and understanding make all the difference during these challenging years.

7

CULTIVATING RELATIONSHIPS

This chapter talks about the sixth part of the 7-Component BALANCE Framework, which is (C): Cultivating relationships. In simple terms, it's about improving communication, making relationships stronger, and deepening intimacy. This chapter emphasizes taking a holistic approach to nurturing connections and building closeness.

JOYCE'S STORY OF REDISCOVERING INTIMACY

After the end of a difficult and coercive marriage, 60-year-old Joyce found herself embarking on a journey through the phases of menopause, facing the unique challenges it presented and its profound impact on her confidence and overall well-being. Joyce focused solely on seeking therapy, rebuilding her life, and embracing the joys of independence and self-care. She had no intention of developing a close relationship.

While enjoying a relaxing yoga retreat in Spain, something amazing happened to her that reignited her feelings of sensuality and longing for closeness. This unexpected encounter sparked a desire within her to seek new opportunities and consider undergoing hormone replacement therapy as a way to manage the symptoms of menopause and regain her energy and vitality.

Joyce's journey of self-discovery and newfound confidence led her to embrace the joys of dating and intimacy, ultimately finding a fulfilling and empowering connection with someone who shared her life stage and outlook.

Her story serves as an inspiring example of the profound impact of menopause on personal growth, resilience, and the potential for new beginnings no matter what life stage you're in.

IMPROVING COMMUNICATION: BREAKING BARRIERS IN SOCIETY

Communication is the lifeline of human connection, shaping our interactions, relationships, and the very fabric of society. Effective communication can bridge gaps, foster inclusivity, and pave the way for a more interconnected and harmonious society—one that acknowledges menopause.

How Improved Communication During Menopause Can Strengthen Relationships, Foster Empathy, and Promote Mutual Support

Menopause can have a huge impact on relationships, and improved communication is the key to navigating these changes. Having open and honest conversations about how you feel physically and emotionally can help strengthen your relationship, build empathy, and provide mutual support. Let's explore some ways better communication can benefit your relationship during menopause (Warwick, 2023; Smith, n.d.):

- **More time to do what they love:** During the menopause stage, children are typically more self-sufficient or are preparing to move out, resulting in couples having more quality time together. It can be a chance for them to enjoy activities like going to a comedy show, flying in a hot air balloon, or simply cherishing each other's company over a cup of coffee.
- **Rekindled love:** Menopause can bring about a stronger bond between partners and a renewed interest in reigniting the romance in the relationship. This might mean showing more affection toward each other, trying out new positions during intercourse, or organizing special date nights.
- **Empathy and understanding:** During menopause, partners need to show a little more compassion and understanding toward each other's experiences. Understanding that menopause is a natural and personal journey for every woman can help partners provide meaningful support to their loved ones.
- **Building a stronger emotional bond:** During menopause, it's good for partners to support and understand each other better by talking openly about their feelings. This can help them act with more compassion toward one another.
- **Healthy lifestyle changes:** Regular exercise and eating well can make menopause symptoms more manageable and boost your mood. You and your partner can encourage each other to make healthy choices together, like going for afternoon walks, engaging in relaxing activities like meditation or yoga, or attending an exercise boot camp together.

- **Practical support:** Assisting with everyday tasks, duties, or menopause symptoms can show that a partner is dedicated to working together and supporting each other. This might involve making practical adjustments, like changing the living space to help with hot flashes or night sweats, or seeking professional guidance if menopause symptoms are greatly impacting well-being and relationships.

When you foster open communication and have mutual support in your relationship, you can navigate the challenges of menopause together while strengthening your relationship.

CHANGE MENOPAUSE FROM A PRIVATE TO A SHARED EXPERIENCE

Talking openly about menopause is important for bringing older and younger generations closer together. Menopause is a normal part of a woman's life that happens to all of us, and when we talk about it openly, we can break down stereotypes, reduce judgment, and create a supportive atmosphere. Here are a few ways that open communication about menopause can help with this (Piccolo, 2023; Shuckburgh, 2023):

- **Reducing wrong perceptions:** When people openly talk about menopause, it helps remove the negative views and misunderstandings surrounding it. By discussing it openly, menopause becomes a normal part of life instead of a shameful topic. This also helps both younger and older generations understand and appreciate the different experiences that come with menopause.
- **Showing compassion and empathy:** Talking about our own experiences and difficulties helps us understand and relate to each other better. When younger people learn

about the physical and emotional effects of menopause, they can show more understanding and support. And when older people understand the unique challenges faced by younger generations, it creates a reciprocal exchange of empathy.

- **Increasing awareness:** Older people can tell younger people about menopause, sharing what they've experienced and what they know. This helps to get rid of false beliefs and disseminate correct information. Younger people can learn about the physical and emotional parts of menopause, which helps them understand and relate better.

- **Navigating healthcare during menopause:** If you want to get the right help and medical treatment, you need to have the confidence to talk openly to your healthcare providers about your menopause. This means discussing any concerns you have, exploring different treatment options, and advocating for personalized care that suits your needs.

- **Encouraging supportive environments:** Having open communication is super important because it helps people feel comfortable asking for help. When it comes to women going through menopause, getting emotional and physical support can make a big difference in how they handle it, so it's awesome when family, friends, and colleagues step up and create a supportive environment by showing some understanding and offering a helping hand.

- **Breaking communication barriers:** Menopause is a topic that can be sensitive, and talking about it openly helps improve communication. When we're open about it, it allows people to share their feelings, worries, and needs without worrying about being judged. By encouraging conversations, we can share information and learn from each other, bridging the gap between different generations.

- **Empowering women:** Open communication allows older women to share their ways of dealing with challenges and staying strong, while younger women can bring in new and different viewpoints and ideas. When we create an environment where everyone feels comfortable expressing themselves, women can work together to question and change the traditional beliefs and expectations around menopause.
- **Promoting health and wellness:** Talking openly about menopause can help improve your health. It's not just for older folks either! Younger generations can start taking charge of their health by learning about preventive measures and making informed choices as they grow older. And hey, even the older generations can benefit from discovering new health practices and gaining fresh wellness perspectives. So let's break the silence and have some menopause chats, shall we?
- **Improving partner communication and intimacy:** Improved communication during menopause can help enhance sexual well-being and closeness by addressing common challenges such as dryness of the vagina, a decreased desire for sex, and worries about body image.
- **Understanding differing viewpoints:** Different cultures have their unique ways of understanding and talking about menopause. It's important to have open conversations that challenge any negative beliefs or stereotypes and promote inclusivity for everyone (*Cultural Perspectives on Menopause*, 2022).

WORKPLACE COMMUNICATION AND MENOPAUSE

Talking openly about menopause at work is extremely important. It fosters a nurturing and inclusive atmosphere that benefits everyone. Better communication can help deal with things like productivity, making necessary adjustments, and providing support for employees going through menopause. Here are some important things to know:

- **Let your voice be heard:** Employers should understand how menopause affects employees' lives and the significance of improving their work-life quality. By promoting open discussions about menopause, employers can gain insight into the different requests of employees going through menopause. This approach can help create a work environment where menopausal employees feel understood and backed by their employer and colleagues ("The 'M' Word," n.d.).
- **Understanding the effect menopause has on women:** Workplaces should have policies that support women going through menopause. They should encourage open communication and provide education about menopause. By doing this, workplaces can better understand and manage the challenges faced by women during menopause and create a more inclusive and supportive environment (Piccolo, 2023).
- **Supporting menopausal employees:** To support women in the workplace who are dealing with the challenges of menopause, the employer must have a workplace policy in place. This policy should explain how the company will support menopausal employees. For example, employers can offer flexible work hours or remote work options, paid

sick leave, and access to on-site health and wellness services for women experiencing menopause.

Open dialogue in the workplace is important for creating a supportive and inclusive environment. If you find yourself in a professional environment, why not be an advocate in the workplace for all women experiencing menopause?

STRENGTHENING RELATIONSHIPS: ENHANCING INTIMATE BONDS DURING MENOPAUSE

I highly recommend that you read this section together with your spouse or partner!

Going through menopause can be tough for couples. The hormonal roller coaster and emotional ups and downs can put a strain on relationships and bring on some stress. But hey, don't worry! It's important to recognize and tackle these challenges head-on to keep your relationship healthy and supportive. Here are some strategies to strengthen your relationship during menopause:

- **Communication is key:** It's important to learn about the physical and emotional symptoms of menopause so that you and your partner can understand each other better and be prepared for mood changes. Don't worry, your partner has your back! Keep those lines of communication open and have honest conversations about hot flashes, mood swings, or low sex drive. It might be a bit uncomfortable, but it's important to address these topics openly.

- **Adjust your expectations:** Menopause can have an impact on your relationship, so it's important to be understanding and adapt your expectations. Find new ways to show affection, manage emotional outbursts, and be open to compromise and negotiation with your partner.
- **Smooth sailing:** Work together to minimize conflicts and misunderstandings. Discuss how to handle sudden impasses or tough situations calmly and respectfully. It's all about finding solutions together.
- **Do things together:** Engage in activities that bring you and your partner closer, like having a special date night, sharing a bedtime routine, or going for a nice walk together. It's all about creating those special moments.
- **Stay connected:** Regularly check in with your partner through phone calls, text messages, or in-person conversations. It's important to maintain that emotional connection and provide support.
- **Improve physical intimacy:** To enhance your physical connection, you can try watching erotic videos, experimenting with different sexual activities, and creating a relaxing atmosphere in the bedroom. It's important to focus on foreplay, talk openly about your comfort levels, and minimize any discomfort during sex. Having honest conversations with your partner about your desires and boundaries is crucial for a satisfying and intimate relationship.
- **Spread the love:** Support your partner by giving compliments, assuring them that you still find them attractive, and acknowledging their efforts in managing menopause symptoms. A little love goes a long way!

- **Seeking help is okay:** If things get tough, don't hesitate to consider couples therapy or counseling. It can be incredibly helpful in navigating the challenges of menopause and strengthening your relationship. You're not alone on this journey!

The Importance of Alone Time and Celebrating Relationship Milestones

Keeping a good relationship means finding the right balance between spending time together and giving each other space. It's important to respect each other's need for alone time and personal space, including doing things on your own. Alone time is pretty important because it helps you stay focused on your own goals, recharge, and become the best version of yourself. So remember, a little "me time" can do wonders for a healthy relationship!

It also allows you to appreciate your partner more from afar, reignite the spark, and make sure you are more present when you're with your partner.

It's important to find a balance between alone time and quality time spent together as a couple. The amount of alone time needed varies from person to person, and it is essential to communicate and respect each other's needs.

Celebrate those special moments and accomplishments in your relationship! It boosts your mood, helps you relax, and keeps you looking on the bright side of things. So raise a toast with your partner to all the good times!

These special moments are not just important tasks to complete, but they are meaningful experiences that have strengthened your relationship, brought you closer together, and deepened your understanding of each other. Some important relationship milestones that are worth celebrating include giving each other cute nicknames, showing affection in public, getting to know each other's friends, making up after an argument, going on trips together, spending your first big holiday together as a couple, and taking part in special rituals that are unique to you as a couple. Celebrating these milestones can help make your relationship stronger and create memories that will last.

FUN ACTIVITIES TO DO WITH YOUR PARTNER

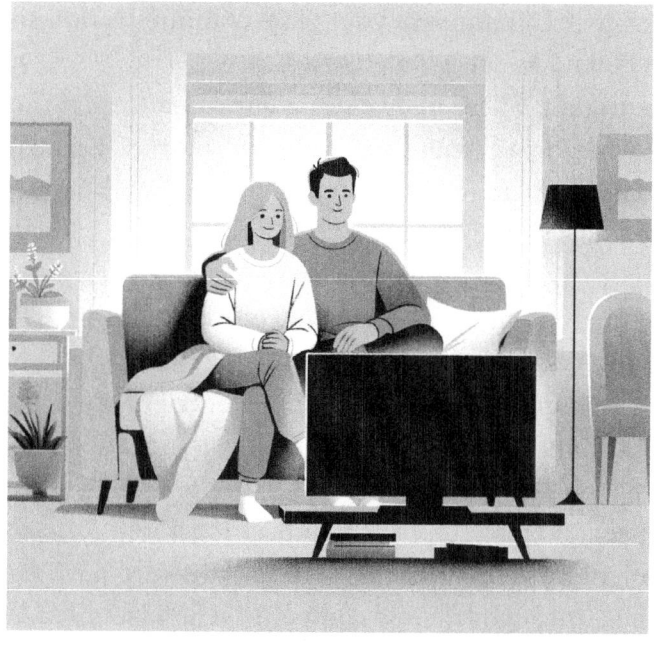

Engaging in activities together can help you strengthen your relationship, create lasting memories, and support each other through the challenges of menopause. It's crucial to find activities that both partners enjoy and that contribute to the overall well-being of your relationship:

- **Walk together:** Going for a walk together is a great way for couples to spend quality time and get some exercise. It lets you enjoy the outdoors, have meaningful conversations, and discover new places. This activity can strengthen your relationship by giving you a chance to connect and bond while also taking care of your health and happiness.
- **Take cooking classes:** Cooking can be a fun bonding activity. It lets you connect while trying out new recipes and discovering different types of food. This shared experience can improve your team communication and help you make special memories.
- **Date nights:** These nights keep your romance alive and give you a break from your everyday routines. Some ideas for date night activities are trying out a new restaurant, watching a movie, going to a concert, or doing something you both love. It's a special time to focus on each other and keep the romantic spark alive in your relationship.
- **Serving your community together:** Volunteering together can strengthen bonds and contribute positively to your community. Finding a cause or organization you both feel passionate about and want to support can help couples connect and make a positive impact together.
- **Game nights:** Game nights are a great way to have fun and connect through friendly competition and laughter. When you play board games, card games, or video games together, it can help you relax and strengthen your relationship as a couple.
- **Get some mutual hobbies:** Exploring new hobbies can add a spark of excitement and rejuvenation to your relationship! Why not try activities like painting, gardening, dancing, or learning a musical instrument

together? They can help you discover shared interests and create amazing new experiences as a couple!

- **Engaging in physical activities:** Engaging in physical activities together is important for managing menopausal symptoms and improving well-being. Options like hiking, biking, swimming, and yoga can help couples stay active and support each other's health.

- **Classes and workshops:** Enrolling in classes or workshops together can be a fun and challenging way to grow as a couple. Art workshops, water aerobics classes, or tap dance lessons provide opportunities for personal growth and shared experiences. Learning something new may eventually develop into a new mutual hobby that both of you can further enjoy together.

- **Weekend getaways:** They're like little escapes for couples where you can relax and have some fun together. It's all about taking a break from the usual stress and just enjoying each other's company. These getaways help you build a stronger connection and make awesome memories that will stick with you. So go ahead and plan your next adventure!

- **Spa days:** Enjoying spa days can be a great way for couples to relax and pamper themselves. You can visit a spa or create a soothing atmosphere at home and treat yourselves to massages, facials, or baths together. This can help you both unwind, relieve stress, and strengthen your bond.

In this chapter, we've talked about surrounding yourself with supportive people and strategies for fostering meaningful relationships. Now that you have the right tools to nurture your relationships, let's talk about embracing menopause with confidence.

8

EMBRACING MENOPAUSE WITH CONFIDENCE

This chapter talks about the very last part of the 7-Component BALANCE Framework, which is all about (E): Embracing menopause with confidence. In Chapter 8, we explore ways to grow personally, boost self-confidence, and celebrate your life experiences.

CELEBRATING THE GIFTS MENOPAUSE BRINGS

You're sitting at your desk, trying to concentrate on your work, but all you can think about is the sudden hot flash that has engulfed your body. It feels like you're standing in the middle of a desert, and the sweat is pouring down your face. Sound familiar? Menopause, with its physical and emotional changes, can leave you feeling overwhelmed and unsure of how to navigate this new phase of life. You need to have the confidence to fully embrace it! Don't let menopause hold you back; let it propel you forward into the best years of your life!

But how do you find gold in a heap of coal? To be able to celebrate your menopause phase, you need to decide which parts of it you are going to embrace. Whether it's your newfound love of yoga, the quiet time of meditation, or meeting with the friends you just made through your online menopause support group, there will be something good to find, embrace, and nurture! Remember, we are as good as our thoughts. Let's focus on the positive side of things! The good news is that once your menopause eventually starts to clear, your newly stable hormone levels can result in improved mental clarity, allowing you to concentrate on personal growth and development.

RECOGNIZING OPPORTUNITIES FOR PERSONAL GROWTH

Menopause can also be an opportunity for personal growth and wisdom. Many women describe positive aspects of menopause, including a time of improved well-being following menopause and relief from dealing with menstruation. It's like entering a new chapter of life where hot flashes become a chance to practice spontaneous fire breathing! Women also acknowledge the potential for personal growth and increased freedom to focus on their own lives.

Remember, this is a transformative phase that offers you a chance for self-reflection and heightened self-awareness. This transition allows you to contemplate your life, values, and priorities, fostering personal discovery and growth. It can be a catalyst for redefining yourself and uncovering new aspects of your identity. Moreover, the absence of menstruation and the wisdom gained during menopause can boost your confidence, self-assurance, and sense of control over various aspects of life. Embracing menopause as a period of self-discovery and transformation can deepen your understanding of your inner dialogue and help reshape your perspective to align with the changes in your body, ultimately enhancing your mental health and overall well-being.

Menopause presents a powerful opportunity to prioritize your health, well-being, and personal development. Welcoming a life-long growth and learning mindset will benefit you throughout your journey.

EMBRACING CHANGE AND EMPOWERING TRANSFORMATION

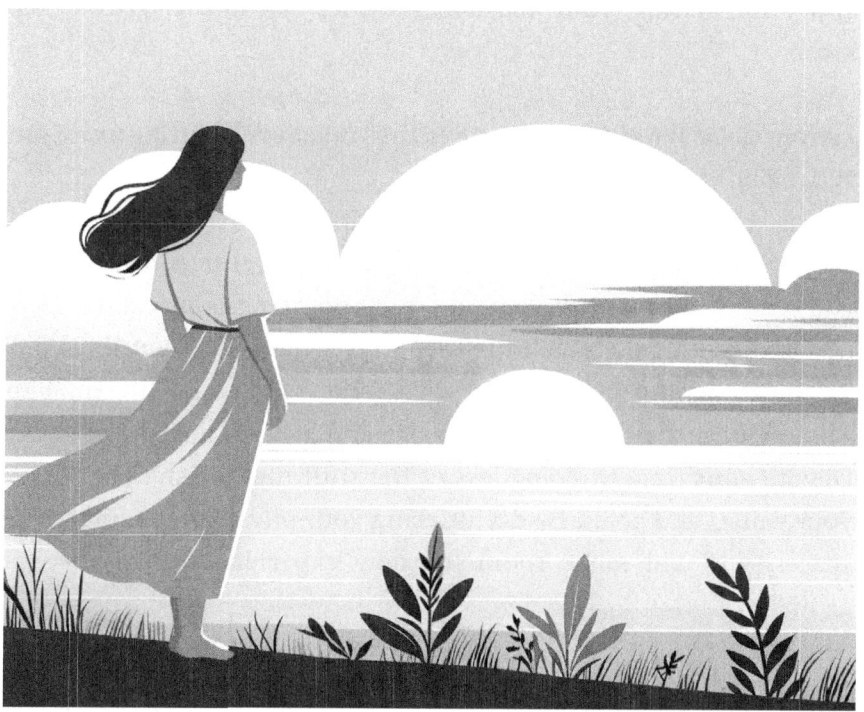

Menopause is a significant phase in a woman's life that brings about various physical and emotional changes. It's a time of transition that can also be an opportunity for personal growth and development. In this section, we'll explore the importance of personal growth during menopause and provide detailed steps and ideas to support women on their journey of self-discovery and empowerment.

Redirecting Your Mindset: Embracing Your Natural Greatness

You were born great. Your growth begins when you redirect your mindset. It is crucial to challenge the societal conditioning that suggests you are not good enough or need to become "more." Real growth involves letting go of these limiting beliefs and embracing the understanding that you are already enough. By recognizing and appreciating your natural greatness, you can grow even more.

Letting Go of What Doesn't Benefit You Anymore: Creating Space for What You Want

You don't grow just because you keep adding things to your life; you only start growing when you start removing things and people that add no value. It's about letting go of what isn't benefiting your life and creating a place for what you want. Take the time to acknowledge that you are adequate and worthy just as you are. Devote your time to doing less of the stuff that doesn't align with your values and goals. By decluttering your physical and emotional spaces, you can make room for new experiences and personal growth.

Discovering Your Natural Strengths: Unleashing Your True Self

Your growth and development should be about becoming more of your real self rather than trying to prove your worth. Take the time to cultivate your natural talents and strengths. Reflect on what brings you pleasure and satisfaction. By embracing your authentic self, you can inspire others and make a positive impact in your personal and professional life.

The Benefits of Personal Growth for Women in Menopause

Engaging in personal growth during menopause offers many benefits for you, including:

- **Improved self-belief:** As you start to recognize your value and let your authentic self shine, your confidence will naturally increase.
- **Greater decision-making abilities:** Your growth enhances your ability to make informed decisions that support your values and goals.
- **Better communication skills:** Your communication with others improves when you develop your self-awareness and self-expression capabilities.
- **Knowing why you're here:** When you grow as a person, your life's purpose becomes clearer to you, and this helps you align your actions to fit your purpose.

Five Powerful Steps to Achieve Personal Growth

To support your growth journey during menopause, consider the following steps:

- **Acknowledging your worth:** Understand that you are valuable and good enough just the way you are, and your worth does not depend on approval or recognition from others.
- **Committing to doing less:** Self-care should be high on your priority list, so focus on activities that align with your values and bring you satisfaction.

- **Sorting what isn't working in your life:** Reflect on your relationships and evaluate your habits and commitments. Let go of those that no longer contribute to your growth and well-being.
- **Determining your innate strengths:** Identify your unique strengths and talents. Leverage them to pursue new opportunities and challenges.
- **Starting a personal growth challenge:** Set specific goals and engage in activities that promote personal growth, such as learning new skills, practicing self-reflection, or seeking new experiences.

More Ideas for Personal Growth

In addition to the steps mentioned above, here are some other personal growth ideas for women in menopause:

- **Use your strengths:** Now that you've identified your innate strengths, you can use them to your advantage. This will build your resilience on your menopausal journey.
- **Build a network:** Surround yourself with supportive and like-minded individuals who can inspire and encourage your personal growth.
- **Find a personal mentor:** Seek guidance from someone who has experienced personal growth and can provide valuable insights and advice.
- **Master the art of being organized:** You need to learn how to be organized to manage your time effectively and create some balance in your life.
- **Learn to say no:** Set boundaries and prioritize your needs by learning to say no to commitments that do not align with your personal growth goals.

CONTINUING THE JOURNEY: LIFELONG LEARNING AND SELF-IMPROVEMENT

Personal growth is an ongoing process that extends beyond menopause. Embrace the mindset of a lifelong learner and continue to seek opportunities for growth and self-improvement. Consider the following practices:

- **Finding passion:** Explore new hobbies and interests that ignite your passion and bring you joy. What have you always dreamed of doing?
- **Developing a vision board:** Imagine your future goals by making a vision board that acts as a visual representation of your growth journey. What would be the first thing you'd add to your board?
- **Reflecting regularly:** Engage in self-reflection to gain insights into your personal growth journey and make necessary adjustments. If you could have a conversation with your future self, what advice would you give you?
- **Beating burnout:** Take care of yourself and set limits to avoid getting exhausted and keep yourself healthy. And guess what? Your secret weapon is laughter, the magical medicine that keeps you strong and ready to face the day!
- **Taking risks:** Step out of your comfort zone and embrace new challenges that push you to grow and expand your horizons. Someone once said, "Fake it till you make it," and even when you are scared, do it anyway.

CELEBRATING YOUR GROWTH: EMBRACING SELF-APPRECIATION AND GRATITUDE

As you start on your growth journey, remember to appreciate yourself and celebrate your progress. Practice self-appreciation and gratitude for the little wins along the way. Take time out for fun and relaxation, try meditation to cultivate mindfulness, travel and explore new places, simplify your life to reduce stress, re-evaluate your goals periodically, volunteer to give back to your community, connect with nature to find solace and inspiration, and celebrate the milestones you achieve.

Starting a gratitude journal can work wonders in embracing self-appreciation and gratitude. By setting aside a few moments each day to reflect on and jot down the things you're grateful for, you can start developing a positive and appreciative mindset. This practice helps shift your focus toward the good things in your life, no matter how small, and nurtures a sense of self-worth and contentment. It's like sprinkling a little extra happiness into your day! Plus, it gives you a chance to celebrate those little wins and milestones, fostering a deeper connection with yourself and promoting a more optimistic outlook on life. So why not give it a try? What are you waiting for? Grab a notebook and begin listing all the things you're grateful for!

Paying it forward can be a great way to celebrate your growth and express gratitude. Sharing your experiences and knowledge and providing support to other women who may be navigating similar paths can create a sense of fulfillment and purpose. Whether it's through mentorship, volunteering, or simply offering a listening ear, contributing to the well-being and success of other women can be a deeply rewarding experience. By paying it forward, you not only acknowledge the value of your growth and learning but also create a positive impact within your community and beyond. This act of generosity and support can further reinforce your self-appreciation and gratitude, fostering a sense of interconnectedness and empowerment among women. So how will you pay it forward to other women and spread the joy of growth and empowerment?

Personal growth is a unique and sometimes lonely journey. Embrace the changes that menopause brings and use this phase as an opportunity for self-discovery, learning, and empowerment. Let this transformative journey guide you on a new adventure, and embrace the joy of blooming into your best self!

BOOSTING YOUR SELF-CONFIDENCE

To boost self-confidence during menopause, practice self-care for the mind and body. Regular exercise enhances mood, reduces stress, and increases energy levels, improving well-being and self-confidence. Focus on a balanced, nutritious diet and adequate sleep for overall health and vitality, positively impacting your self-esteem and confidence. Engage in physical activities like yoga, swimming, or walking to promote health, lift your mood, manage weight, and improve body image and self-confidence. Instead of thinking negatively, try using positive statements to boost your mood. Be kind and understanding toward yourself, and take time to acknowledge and celebrate even the smallest accomplishments. This will help you develop a positive inner dialogue and increase your self-confidence. Additionally, it's important to be aware that hormonal changes and physical symptoms experienced during menopause, such as changes in skin and hair loss, can also affect self-esteem.

Several strategies can help you develop self-confidence during this phase:

- **Self-care and physical well-being:** Don't forget to treat yourself like the superstar you are by nourishing your body, staying active, and catching those ZZZs! It's all about that self-care groove!

- **Replace self-criticism with mindful thoughts:** Be mindful of your internal thoughts and confront any pessimistic self-talk. Replace self-critical thoughts with positive affirmations and reminders of your strengths and accomplishments. Remember, you're a superstar in your unique way!
- **Treat yourself with compassion:** Be kind to yourself and practice self-compassion. Accept that menopause is a natural part of life and that it's normal to experience a range of emotions during this time. Extend yourself the same level of kindness and empathy that you would offer to a dear friend.
- **Find support:** Surround yourself with a supportive network of friends, family members, or support groups who can provide encouragement and understanding. Sharing experiences with others going through similar journeys can help foster a sense of belonging and boost confidence.
- **Set realistic goals:** Break down bigger goals into smaller, achievable steps. And hey, don't forget to celebrate each accomplishment along the way! It's like giving yourself a little confidence and motivation boost as you keep moving forward.
- **Embrace your growth:** Menopause is a phase of life during which women go through changes. Don't focus on the negative changes; instead, make a list of what is good about this phase and embrace this time as a growth opportunity. Use the good to build an even better life.
- **Seek professional help if needed:** If feelings of low self-confidence don't go away after a short while or affect your daily life, consider getting support from a healthcare professional or therapist. They can provide guidance, coping strategies, and additional resources to help you

navigate this phase with confidence. You don't have to face it alone—there are experts out there ready to lend a helping hand and a listening ear!

POSITIVE SELF-TALK AFFIRMATIONS

Here are some positive affirmations for women in menopause to boost confidence:

- I am strong, resilient, and capable of dealing with the changes of menopause.
- I embrace and celebrate the wisdom and experience that menopause brings.
- I am worthy of acceptance, love, and respect from others.
- I am beautiful inside and out, and my worth is not defined by societal standards.
- I have complete control over my thoughts and emotions, and I consciously choose to direct my focus toward positivity and self-care.
- I am grateful for the unique qualities and strengths that make me who I am.
- I am resilient, capable, and worthy of achieving my goals and dreams.
- I trust my body's ability to adapt and find balance during this transitional phase.
- I am proud of the woman I have become and the challenges I have overcome.
- I choose to prioritize my well-being and make self-care a priority.
- I release self-judgment and embrace self-compassion and kindness during this time.
- I am open to new possibilities and opportunities for growth, learning, and personal development.

- I honor my needs and boundaries and confidently communicate them to others.
- I am surrounded by a supportive network of loved ones who uplift and empower me.
- I have confidence in my ability to make choices that correspond with my values and needs.

Feel free to choose the affirmations that you find fitting and make them a part of your daily routine. Repeat them to yourself regularly in the mirror, especially during moments when you need a confidence boost. Remember, positive self-affirmations can have a powerful impact on your mindset and self-perception during menopause.

ELEVATING BEAUTY HABITS FOR MENOPAUSAL SKIN: EMBRACING CONFIDENCE, COMFORT, HYGIENE, AND GROOMING

Take care of your physical appearance by creating a skincare routine specifically designed for menopausal skin. This routine should address common issues such as dryness, sagging, and wrinkles. By targeting these concerns, you can maintain the health and vitality of your skin during this stage of life.

Taking Good Care of Your Looks: Skincare Tips for Menopausal Skin and Dressing to Feel Fabulous!

When it comes to looking your best during menopause, it's important to give your skin some extra tender loving care. That means crafting a skincare routine that targets those pesky issues like dryness, sagging, and wrinkles. By doing so, you'll maintain a vibrant image.

But that's not all! Wearing clothing that makes you feel assured and comfortable is a game-changer. When you dress in outfits that boost your self-esteem, not only will you look amazing, but you'll also rock that positive mindset.

Oh, and let's not forget about good hygiene and grooming habits. These little daily rituals of cleanliness and self-care make a big difference in keeping you looking well-groomed and presentable. So remember to pamper yourself a bit because you deserve it!

Other Self-Care Tips During Menopause

- **Make bedtime a little comfier:** Invest in comfortable, breathable pajamas that help control your body temperature. Get yourself a satin pillowcase—it stays cool and helps your skin resist the formation of wrinkles.
- **Enjoy a cup of healthy tea:** For some of us, a warm cup of tea fixes almost everything. Enjoy a calming, soothing experience with teas that contain special herbs known to help balance hormones and ease menopause symptoms. You can explore black cohosh and dong quai teas, known to support hormonal balance. Also, try tea blends with red clover, sage, and licorice root as they have been traditionally used to reduce hot flashes, night sweats, and mood swings.
- **Menopause fitness attire:** Shop for workout clothes that are both stylish and comfortable. Opt for moisture-wicking fabrics.
- **Snack on healthy options:** Choose nutrient-dense snacks that provide long-lasting energy.
- **Natural cooling products:** Cooling sprays and pads are designed to provide instant relief from hot flashes and night sweats. Try it out!

MENOPAUSE: ITS RELATIONSHIP WITH YOUR SKIN AND HAIR

Skin problems are caused by your declining estrogen levels. This affects your body's natural collagen production, resulting in more wrinkles, fine lines, and overall dryness. Lack of hydration is a key skin concern during menopause. Collagen helps keep your skin hydrated, and once the collagen in your body declines, your skin begins its journey through the desert. But hey, don't worry! Plenty of skincare products and routines are out there to help us keep our skin glowing and feeling fabulous (*Caring for Your Skin in Menopause*, 2023).

During menopause, it's common for women to experience changes in their hair and skin. These changes can include hair becoming thinner, drier, and less shiny as well as differences in skin texture. To combat these changes, skincare strategies include using peptides to spur the production of collagen and reduce fine lines and wrinkles. Retinol also helps curb the appearance of wrinkles and fine lines. Other skincare strategies include using sunscreen daily for skin protection and wrinkle reduction and moisturizing your skin regularly to combat age-related moisture loss. Products with hyaluronic acid and ceramides can improve hydration and moisture retention. If you want something to help restore your body's hormonal balance, peptide therapy is something you can consider as it can also help alleviate menopause symptoms (*Female Peptide Therapy*, n.d.). Patch testing for sensitive skin concerns can be a valuable aspect of your skincare journey when trying out new products.

You can manage dark spots by using topical antioxidants like vitamin C, and don't skimp on sunscreen! Prevention is the best cure. Protecting your skin from the sun's rays is important, especially if you have a lighter skin tone. Use a broad-spectrum sunscreen to prevent extensive skin pigmentation (Petrullo, 2023). What's your go-to sunscreen for keeping your skin safe and sound?

When you go through menopause, you may grow more facial hair because your estrogen levels decrease. It's a good idea to talk to a doctor about this issue. They can consider hair removal therapies like laser. Another thing to think about during menopause is acne treatment. Hormonal changes can cause more oil on your skin and therefore more pimples. Control breakouts and keep your skin healthy by using cleansers containing glycolic acid or salicylic acid (Gallagher, 2022).

Hormonal shifts and sun damage can lead to pigmentation issues, such as melasma or chloasma. These problems occur when elevated estrogen and progesterone levels cause your skin to make more melanin. Other factors that result in your skin creating more melanin can be skin inflammation and the use of, for example, contraceptives. When directly exposed to bright sunlight, your skin will be like a magnet for attracting dark spots (Tamira Scientific Committee, 2023). To get rid of dark spots, you can use skincare products that contain antioxidants such as vitamin C.

Skincare needs vary from person to person, so it may require some trial and error to find what works best for you. If you have sensitive skin, it is recommended that you perform a patch test before trying new products (Mayer, 2022).

Beautiful Hair and Skin: Your Ultimate Tip Box

Now, let's recap what we've discussed and explore some straightforward tips to maintain healthier hair and skin. There are specific steps you can take to care for your skin and hair:

- Stay hydrated by drinking plenty of water daily.
- Make sure you sleep enough every night.
- Relieve an irritated scalp with a scalp-refreshing shampoo.
- If you smoke, try to stop.
- Drink less alcohol and manage your stress levels.
- Boost hair health by adding natural ingredients like argan oil and rosemary essential oil to your conditioner or by buying products that contain these ingredients.
- Search for skincare lines that specifically cater to women in this phase of life.
- Use peptides and retinol to reduce the appearance of fine lines and wrinkles (Deanna, 2022; Burcham & Nouril, 2024).
- Combat dryness by using products with ingredients like hyaluronic acid, glycerin, and ceramides to help the skin retain moisture (*Caring for Your Skin in Menopause*, 2023).
- Methods such as threading, plucking, laser hair removal, shaving, topical creams, and electrolysis are available to manage facial hair. However, it's important to talk to your doctor to rule out any underlying health issues first. Sometimes medication may be prescribed (Mayer, 2022).
- Treat acne during menopause with cleansers containing salicylic or glycolic acid. Retinol cleansers may also be helpful for women without dry skin.
- Mitigate discoloration by using a topical antioxidant with vitamin C and wearing broad-spectrum sunscreen daily.
- A simple skincare routine example for menopause and beyond includes washing your face with a mild cleanser, using a moisturizer with ceramides and hyaluronic acid, applying sunscreen with an SPF of 30 or higher, and using an antiaging product containing peptides at night.

Menopause-Friendly Skincare Products

Skincare products that are suitable for menopausal women usually have ingredients that can help with the specific problems that come with menopausal skin, like dryness, dullness, and sensitivity. Some of the usual ingredients found in menopause-friendly skincare products are (Hogan, 2022; *8 Ingredients to Glowing Skin During Menopause*, 2022; Shotter, 2022):

- **Vitamin C:** The antioxidants in vitamin C help reduce inflammation and boost collagen production, which is great for your skin.
- **Retinol:** This is a strong ingredient that helps reduce signs of aging. It is commonly found in skincare products that are suitable for menopausal women.
- **Niacinamide:** This is a type of vitamin B3 that can help decrease redness often linked to hot flashes.
- **Hyaluronic acid:** This ingredient helps retain moisture in the skin.
- **Ceramides:** These are lipids that help maintain the protective activity of your skin.
- **Omega fatty acids:** Omega-3 and omega-6 fatty acids help support skin health.
- **Glycerin:** This is a natural moisturizer.
- **Peptides:** This helps support collagen and elastin production.

Not-So-Menopause-Friendly Skincare Ingredients

Some ingredients to avoid in skincare products during menopause include (Chow & Mahalingaiah, 2016; Shotter, 2022; *Caring for Your Skin in Menopause*, 2023; Mayer, 2022):

- Fragrances can be irritating to menopausal skin, which may already be more sensitive due to hormonal changes. Instead, try to choose skincare products scented with natural essential oils.
- Alcohol can be drying and may worsen the dryness that often comes with menopausal skin.
- Menopausal skin is more delicate, so using harsh exfoliants can cause irritation and damage the skin's protective barrier.
- Retinoids can be helpful for some menopausal skin concerns, but they can also irritate your skin. Use them cautiously and with guidance from a dermatologist.
- Try not to use products that contain phthalates or parabens, chemicals commonly found in skincare products that are linked to potential health risks.
- Cleansers that deplete the skin's own oils might exacerbate dry skin. It's better to choose gentle hydrating cleansers.
- Sulfates can be drying and may worsen the dryness and sensitivity that often come with menopausal skin. It's best to avoid skincare products that contain sulfates.
- Mineral oils like paraffin wax and petroleum jelly simply create a layer on the skin. They can't be absorbed because their molecules are too big, and they don't have any nourishing properties since they are derived from petroleum. Instead, you can use vegetable oils, which can be absorbed by the skin and provide additional nutrients for healing and moisturizing.

REMEMBER TO CELEBRATE "YOU"

Let's review: Menopause is a big deal, but it's also a time to feel empowered. It's a chance to celebrate your body's strength and resilience, which has carried you through all sorts of challenges and experiences. Instead of getting caught up in the changes and potential difficulties, let's embrace this new chapter. How will you celebrate your journey through menopause?

Now, when it comes to celebrating menopause, there are plenty of fun options. You could have dinner parties, book club gatherings, coffee meet-ups, mini retreats, outdoor adventures, or even spa days. These events give you a chance to connect with others and find support during this transformative time. It's an opportunity to reflect on the beauty of your body and the amazing experiences it has allowed you to have. What kind of menopause celebration sounds most exciting to you?

Of course, self-care is also super important during menopause. You need to listen to your body and show it some love. That means engaging in activities like exercise, eating a nutritious diet, and staying cool to help you navigate the changes that come with menopause. What's your favorite way to practice self-care during this special time?

Make it a point to go out fully dressed up with flawless makeup and feel yourself shine.

Each person's menopausal experience is unique, so it's important to be adaptable and open to experimentation when it comes to self-care. By celebrating menopause and prioritizing self-care, you can approach this new phase of life with a sense of empowerment and positivity. Remember when we were teenagers and going through puberty? It was like a special rite of passage into adulthood. Well, now that we're experiencing menopause, it's bringing us even more wisdom and opportunities to make our lives better in the future. We've put in a lot of hard work to get to this point, so let's celebrate together because we deserve it!

BONUS: YOUR PERSONAL MENOPAUSE JOURNEY

The stories of the women we read about in this book show us how strong and resilient women are during menopause. Despite facing different symptoms and challenges, some of these women turned their experiences into testimonies that educate women about the realities of perimenopause and menopause. Their journeys remind us that each woman's experience is unique, and by listening to our bodies and supporting each other, we can navigate this stage of life with grace and determination.

YOUR PERSONAL MENOPAUSE JOURNEY

As we come to the end of our journey together, I would like to thank you with a special gift: a bonus chapter to recap what we've discussed and learned on our voyage and to help you plan for the future. But your journey doesn't end here. I want to encourage you to delve deeper, read and talk, and find out as much about menopause as you possibly can. And remember, make the circle bigger! Build your tribe of women who are going through the same phase in their lives right now.

As you go through menopause, it's important to embrace this new phase of life with purpose and a clear plan for your physical and emotional well-being. This special chapter will help you set meaningful goals and create a personalized menopause plan to guide you on your journey. By celebrating your life experience and embracing the challenges and opportunities that come with this stage, you can have a positive and fulfilling menopause experience.

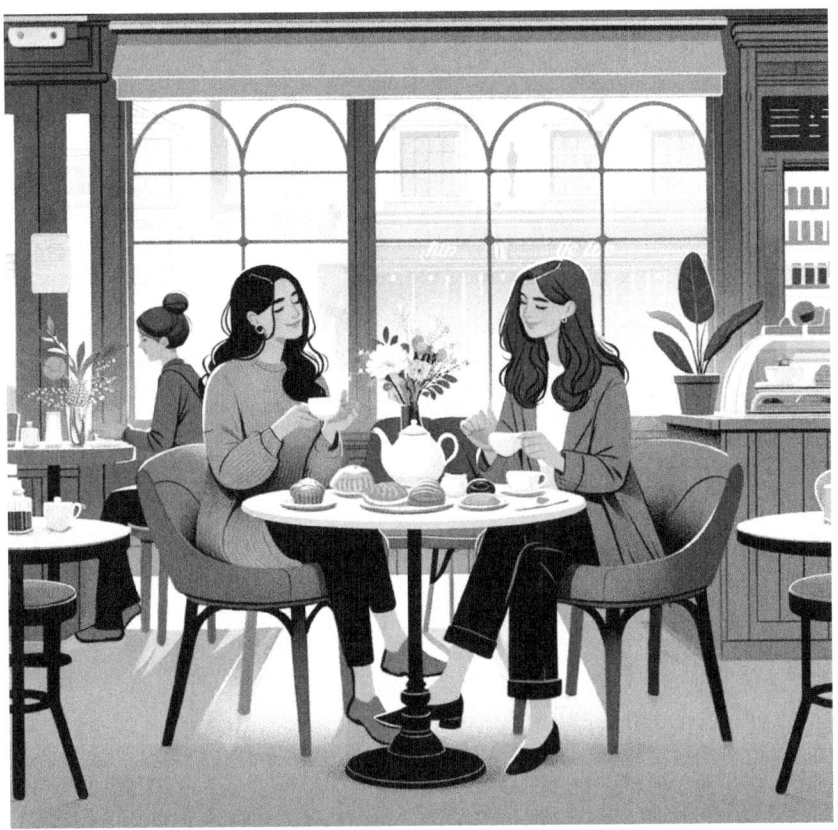

CELEBRATING MENOPAUSE PLANNER

Coffee Meet-ups:

With	Where	When

Other activities (dinner parties, book club, mini retreats, outdoor adventures, spa days...):

With	Where	When

Online communities you want to join:

Group name	Platform or website link	What it offers you

These gatherings provide an opportunity to connect with your community as well as give and find support. It's a chance to reflect on the beauty of your body and the experiences it has enabled you to have. Embracing menopause as a positive life event can help you approach this new phase of life with a sense of empowerment and positivity.

SCHEDULE REGULAR CHECKUPS

My last checkup was on	My next checkup will be on

SYMPTOM CHECKER

Symptom	Yes/No
• **Hot flashes:** Do you find yourself encountering abrupt and intense sensations of heat, frequently accompanied by perspiration and flushed skin?	
• **Night sweats:** Do you often find yourself waking up all sweaty in the middle of the night?	
• **Irregular periods:** Have you noticed changes in the regularity or duration of your menstrual cycles?	
• **Sleep issues:** Are you struggling to sleep when you close your eyes, or do you wake up throughout the night for no reason at all?	
• **Mood changes:** Have you experienced mood swings, irritability, or feelings of anxiety or depression?	
• **Vaginal dryness:** Have you noticed a decrease in vaginal lubrication or discomfort during intercourse?	
• **Decreased libido:** Have you experienced a decline in sexual desire or interest?	
• **Weight gain:** Have you gained weight, especially around the abdomen, despite no significant changes in diet or exercise?	
• **Constantly tired:** Do you lack energy and feel exhausted all the time?	
• **Memory issues:** Have you noticed difficulties with memory or concentration?	
• **Joint pain:** Are you experiencing increased joint pain or stiffness?	
• **Headaches:** Have you been experiencing more frequent or stronger headaches lately?	

• **Breast tenderness:** Have you experienced increased sensitivity or tenderness in your breasts?	
• **Hair changes:** Have you noticed changes in the texture, thickness, or pattern of your hair?	
• **Skin changes:** Have you observed changes in your skin, such as dryness, thinning, or more wrinkles?	
• **Urinary changes:** Have you noticed changes in urinary frequency, urgency, or incontinence?	
• **Digestive issues:** Have you experienced changes in digestion, such as bloating or changes in bowel habits?	
• **Heart palpitations:** Have you felt irregular or rapid heartbeats?	
Other:	

SETTING GOALS FOR YOUR WELL-BEING

As you create your personalized menopause plan, it's essential to set meaningful goals that align with your values and priorities. Some goals to consider include

- Prioritizing self-care and physical health.
- Strengthening your social support network.
- Exploring new hobbies or passions.
- Enhancing your emotional well-being.
- Learning more about menopause and its effects on your body.

By setting specific, measurable, and achievable goals, you can confidently navigate the distinctive journey of menopause. Every woman's menopause experience is different, so be open to experimentation and adaptability as you work toward your goals.

My personalized menopause goals

Embracing your personal menopause journey requires self-aware-ness, self-care, and a willingness to adapt. But don't fret—you've got this!

CONCLUSION

Congratulations on completing this transformative book! Throughout the chapters, you've delved into the 7-Component BALANCE Framework, gaining valuable insights and practical tools to navigate menopause with confidence and optimism. As you reflect on your journey, it's important to recognize the profound impact of the lessons you've learned and the positive changes that lie ahead.

EMBRACING MENOPAUSE AS A NEW BEGINNING

Menopause is not the end of a chapter but the beginning of a new and meaningful stage of life. You can mitigate the effects of menopausal symptoms by redefining it as a positive milestone and embracing the wonder and strength of your body that has carried you through various experiences. It's a time to celebrate the freedom from menstrual cycles and the opportunities for personal growth and fulfillment.

Self-Care: A Foundation for Well-Being

The self-care tips shared by women who have experienced menopause emphasize the importance of being gentle with yourself, listening to your body, and prioritizing your own needs. By adopting healthy nutrition, staying active, and practicing gratitude, you can nurture your physical and emotional well-being. Menopause is an opportunity to reconnect with yourself and practice much-needed self-care, setting the stage for a fulfilling and vibrant future.

A Positive Mindset: The Key to a Fulfilling Menopause Journey

The attitude with which you approach menopause can have a tremendous impact on your experience. By focusing on the positive aspects of growing older, gaining freedom, and the possibilities of personal development, you can embrace menopause with optimism and resilience. Menopause is a time of choice and empowerment, and your positive mindset will guide you toward a fulfilling and enriching journey.

Celebrating Your Journey

As you move forward, consider celebrating this significant milestone in your life. Whether it's through coffee meet-ups, dinner parties, or outdoor adventures, celebrating menopause is an opportunity to honor the strength and resilience of women and create a supportive community. By celebrating menopause, you are not only embracing your journey but also inspiring and supporting women from all walks of midlife.

Looking Ahead: A Future Filled With Purpose

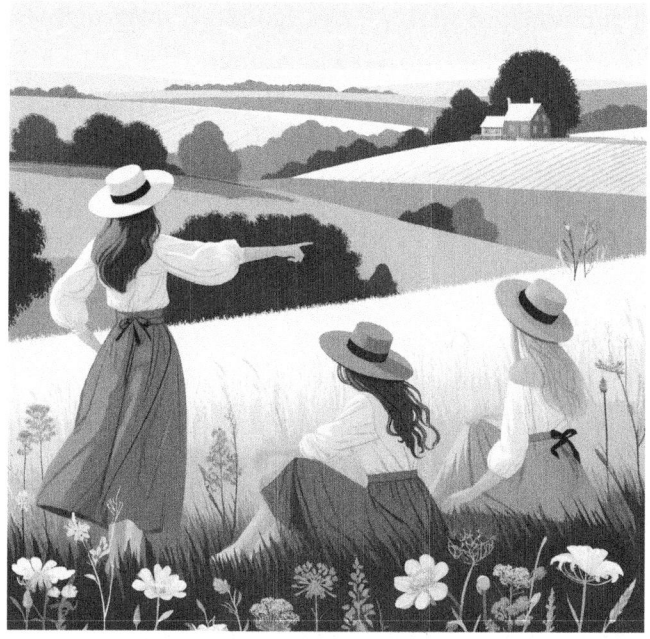

As you enter the years after menopause, it's important to know that this is a time of freedom, personal growth, and pursuing your passions and purpose. The information and skills you've gained from this book will be like a guide, helping you navigate toward a future that's full of energy and satisfaction. By empowering yourself, building meaningful connections, and living with purpose, you're ready to embrace this new phase of life with confidence and elegance.

As you've turned the last page of this book, I hope that you've gained valuable insights and practical tools to help you navigate your menopause journey with confidence and grace. Don't worry if you feel you cannot practice all the ideas here. Imagine you have received a toolbox as a gift—just choose and use whatever tools suit you, and you can even share them with others.

I would like to know what you think about the book and how it has affected your understanding and experience of menopause. By sharing your journey with others, you can help increase awareness, offer support, and motivate women from all backgrounds. Feel free to leave a review. Your feedback is extremely valuable to other women seeking information about menopause, and I am excited to hear from you too. Together, we can build a caring community that empowers women to flourish during menopause and beyond.

In closing, your menopause journey is a testament to your strength and resilience. By integrating the lessons and insights from this book into your life, you are equipped to navigate the distinctive challenges and opportunities of menopause with a sense of purpose. Embrace this valuable and meaningful stage of life, knowing that you have the tools and inner strength to thrive. Here's to a future packed with purpose, happiness, and empowerment!

SUSTAINING THE MOMENTUM AND SHARE THE WEALTH OF WISDOM

Now that you've mastered your menopause, it's time to guide others seeking the same triumphs. Your journey doesn't end here —it continues as you pass on the torch of knowledge to fellow women.

By simply sharing your honest thoughts about this book on Amazon.com, you're not just leaving a review; you're lighting the way for others searching for insights on menopause. Your passion becomes the beacon that helps kindred spirits navigate their path with confidence.

Thank you for being the bridge to knowledge. The world of Menopausal women thrives when we generously share our experiences, and your contribution is invaluable in keeping the flame alive.

Will you take 60 seconds to help another woman? Scan the QR code below to leave your review on Amazon.com:

If you purchased the book from another Amazon site, you can go to "Your Orders" in your account, choose the book, and click "Write a product review".

With sincere gratitude from my heart for joining in the mission to spread wisdom and make the world a better-informed place,

Your partner in knowledge sharing,

Hera Bennett

ABOUT THE AUTHOR

Hera Bennett is a vibrant and insightful woman in her 50s and a mother of two daughters. She was a breastfeeding mother and certified consultant who helped many mothers breastfeed successfully. Now she is supporting women in menopause as a continuation of her commitment to empower women.

Drawing upon her background working in women's health and wellness as well as extensive research, the author provides invaluable guidance to women facing the challenges of menopause. Hera is deeply committed to dismantling the stigma surrounding menopause and reshaping the narrative around this natural phase of life. Through her heartfelt books, she offers practical advice, evidence-based information, and emotional support that aims to ease the physical and emotional transitions during menopause.

She is a dynamic and compassionate author dedicated to empowering women who are navigating the transformative journey of menopause. Her warm and empathetic approach resonates with readers, making her a trusted voice in the realm of menopause literature. Through her books and advocacy, she encourages and inspires women to seek holistic well-being during menopause. Her mission is to empower women to embrace this phase of life with confidence and grace.

Updates From the Author and a Chance for a FREE Book

Let's celebrate menopause together! Join our mailing list and be the first to know about new upcoming books and receive updates and newsletters. You may even receive a FREE book!

To join our mailing list, email:

MenopauseWellnessBook@gmail.com

P.S. - Please add this address to your contact list to avoid emails going to the spam folder. Watch your inbox for updates and to see if you'll be receiving a FREE book!

ALSO BY THE AUTHOR

If you find *The Ultimate Guide to Menopause* helpful in your menopause journey, consider reading the official workbook and other published and upcoming books from Hera Bennett. Join our mailing list to receive updates whenever a new book is launched.

MENOPAUSE WELLNESS SERIES

The Ultimate Guide to Menopause:

7 Easy Steps to Achieve Symptom Relief, Weight Loss, and Holistic Wellness to Confidently Embark on Your Stress-Free Journey

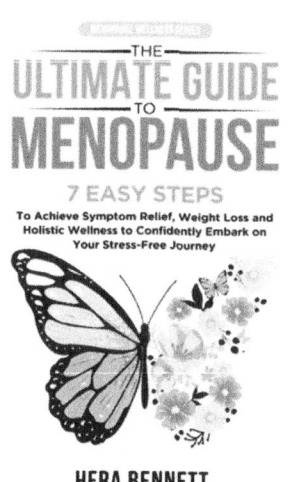

The Ultimate Guide to Menopause Workbook:

7 Easy Steps in Action: Your Tailored Plan to Achieve Symptom Relief, Weight Loss, and Holistic Wellness

The Ultimate Guide to Menopause Anti-Aging:

7 Easy Steps for Skincare and Vitality to Confidently Look and Feel Younger

≈

The Ultimate Guide to Menopause Gut Health:

7 Easy Steps to Restore Your Gut to Improve Digestion, Balance Hormones, Strengthen Immunity and Optimize Well-Being

≈

The Ultimate Guide to Menopause Inner Child Healing:

7 Easy Steps to Overcome Trauma, Rediscover Yourself, and Reclaim Your Life

≈

PARENTING PERSPECTIVES SERIES

Natural Parenting Hacks:

Raising Happy and Healthy Baby in a Loving, No-cry and Holistic Way. Quick Tips for New Parents to Get it Right From The Start

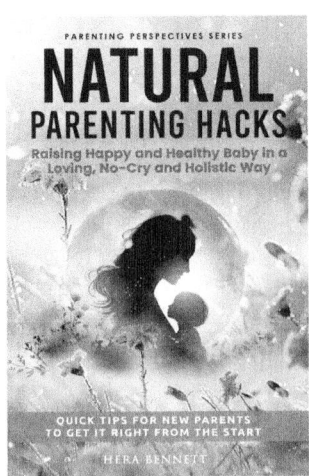

ABOUT THE ARTIST

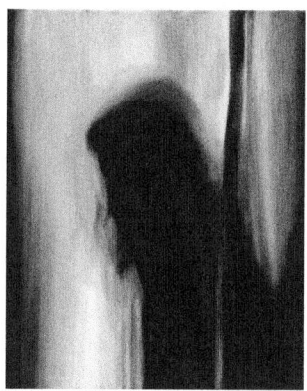

Ngai Ning Yu is a young artist based in London. Her recent work explores the concept of 'the home' with atmospheric paintings depicting interior spaces where traces of human presence are felt. The award-winning artist studied Fine Art Painting at the University of Arts London, and her artworks have been exhibited internationally in prestigious galleries and art fairs.

Please visit www.ngaining.com or scan the QR code to contact the artist.

@NGAINING_ARTIST

REFERENCES

Abramson, A. (2022, November 1). Meditation techniques to help with menopause symptoms. *Stripes.* https://iamstripes.com/blogs/mental-health/meditation-techniques-to-help-with-menopause-symptoms

Abramson, A. (2023, January 9). What is the right balance of strength training to cardio? *The New York Times.* https://www.nytimes.com/2023/01/03/well/move/strength-training-cardio-exercise.html

American Heart Association. (2004, November 18). *High doses of vitamin E supplements do more harm than good.* ScienceDaily. www.sciencedaily.com/releases/2004/11/041116233312.htm

American Heart Association Editorial Staff. (n.d.). *Estrogen, hormone therapy and menopause.* Go Red for Women. https://www.goredforwomen.org/en/know-your-risk/menopause/estrogen-and-hormone-therapy

Ames, H. (2023, November 8). *What is dong quai, and what are its uses?* Medical News Today. https://www.medicalnewstoday.com/articles/dong-quai#dosage

Anderson, C. A. M., Cobb, L. K., Miller, E. R., III, Woodward, M., Hottenstein, A., Chang, A. R., Mongraw-Chaffin, M., White, K., Charleston, J., Tanaka, T., Thomas, L., & Appel, L. J. (2015). Effects of a behavioral intervention that emphasizes spices and herbs on adherence to recommended sodium intake: results of the SPICE randomized clinical trial. *The American journal of clinical nutrition, 102*(3), 671–679. https://doi.org/10.3945/ajcn.114.100750

Appleby, R. (n.d.). *Homeopathy and menopause - Top 5 homeopathic remedies.* My Second Spring. https://mysecondspring.ie/menopause-treatments-and-therapies/homeopathy-and-menopause

Ask the Doctors. (2021, September 29). *Many women have cognition issues during menopause.* UCLA Health. https://www.uclahealth.org/news/many-women-have-cognition-issues-during-menopause

Atkinson, D. (2020, September 24). *A fitness expert's guide to the best 12-week fitness plans for prime women.* Prime Women. https://primewomen.com/wellness/fitness/12-week-plan/

Balzer, D. (2021, May 3). *Mayo Clinic minute: Lifestyle changes to manage menopause symptoms.* Mayo Clinic News Network. https://newsnetwork.mayoclinic.org/discussion/mayo-clinic-minute-lifestyle-changes-to-manage-menopause-symptoms/

The benefits of evening primrose oil during menopause. (n.d.). ReNue Pharmacy.

https://renuerx.com/nutraceuticals/the-benefits-of-evening-primrose-oil-during-menopause/

BetterHelp Editorial Team. (2023, December 9). *How to foster a healthy mind-body connection*. BetterHelp. https://www.betterhelp.com/advice/general/what-is-the-mind-body-connection/

Breus, M. J. (2018, July 12). 4 awesome mind-body therapies for menopause and sleep. *Psychology Today*. https://www.psychologytoday.com/us/blog/sleep-newzzz/201807/4-awesome-mind-body-therapies-menopause-and-sleep

Burcham, C., & Nouril, P. (2024, January 16). *Menopause skincare: Follow these 6 steps to enhance your complexion*. Women's Health. https://www.womenshealthmag.com/uk/beauty/skin/a35778400/menopause-skincare/

Burger, H. G., Dudley, E. C., Robertson, D. M., & Dennerstein, L. (2002). Hormonal changes in the menopause transition. *Recent progress in hormone research*, *57*(1), 257–275. https://doi.org/10.1210/rp.57.1.257

Caring for your skin in menopause. (2023, November 20). American Academy of Dermatology Association. https://www.aad.org/public/everyday-care/skin-care-secrets/anti-aging/skin-care-during-menopause

Cefaratti-Bertin, S. (2023, October 17). *Managing menopause: Mind-body solutions for hot flashes, sleep and well-being*. Baylor University Media and Public Relations. https://news.web.baylor.edu/news/story/2023/managing-menopause-mind-body-solutions-hot-flashes-sleep-and-well-being

Chow, E. T., & Mahalingaiah, S. (2016). Cosmetics use and age at menopause: is there a connection? *Fertility and sterility*, *106*(4), 978–990. https://doi.org/10.1016/j.fertnstert.2016.08.020

Chung, D. J., Kim, H. Y., Park, K. H., Jeong, K. A., Lee, S. K., Lee, Y. I., Hur, S. E., Cho, M. S., Lee, B. S., Bai, S. W., Kim, C. M., Cho, S. H., Hwang, J. Y., & Park, J. H. (2007). Black cohosh and St. John's wort (GYNO-Plus) for climacteric symptoms. *Yonsei medical journal*, *48*(2), 289–294. https://doi.org/10.3349/ymj.2007.48.2.289

Common symptoms. (2014, May 28). Red Hot Mamas. https://redhotmamas.org/menopause-a-z/common-symptoms

A complete guide to diluting essential oils. (n.d.). Anveya. https://www.anveya.com/blogs/top-tips/a-complete-guide-to-diluting-essential-oils

Cordani, A. (n.d.). 'My menopause clashed with my daughter's puberty.' My Menopause Centre. https://www.mymenopausecentre.com/menopause-stories/my-menopause-clashed-with-my-daughters-puberty/

Coveney, P. (2013). *Menopause yoga with Petra Coveney*. Menopause Yoga. https://www.menopause-yoga.com/

Crandall, C. J., Mehta, J. M., & Manson, J. E. (2023). Management of menopausal symptoms. *JAMA*, *329*(5), 405. https://doi.org/10.1001/jama.2022.24140

Crowther, P. (n.d.). *Menopausal signs you might need more vitamin E*. Penny Crowther Mid Life Nutrition. https://nutritionistlondon.co.uk/menopause-help-vitamin-e/

Cultural perspectives on menopause. (2022, August 30). Continence Foundation of Australia. https://www.continence.org.au/news/cultural-perspectives-menopause

CureJoy Editorial. (2017, December 18). *Tai chi moves for beginners: 7 basic steps*. CureJoy. https://curejoy.com/content/tai-chi-moves-for-beginners/

Dairy. (n.d.). Harvard T.H. Chan School of Public Health. https://www.hsph.harvard.edu/nutritionsource/dairy/

Davidson, K. (2020, August 20). *Red clover: Benefits, uses, and side effects*. Healthline. https://www.healthline.com/nutrition/red-clover

Davis, C., Bryan, J., Hodgson, J., & Murphy, K. (2015). Definition of the Mediterranean diet; A literature review. *Nutrients, 7*(11), 9139–9153. https://doi.org/10.3390/nu7115459

Davis, J. L. (n.d.). *Tips to reduce stress in women over 50*. WebMD. https://www.webmd.com/women/women-over-50-tips-to-reduce-stress

Deanna. (2022, May 19). *The wonders of peptides for menopause*. Well & Worthy Life. https://wellandworthylife.com/peptides-for-menopause/

Does mindfulness help with menopause? (2023, June 12). Balance by Newton Health. https://www.balance-menopause.com/menopause-library/does-mindfulness-help-with-menopause/

Dong quai. (n.d.). Mount Sinai Health System. https://www.mountsinai.org/health-library/herb/dong-quai

Dong quai: Purported benefits, side effects & more. (2023, August 23). Memorial Sloan Kettering Cancer Center. https://www.mskcc.org/cancer-care/integrative-medicine/herbs/dong-quai

Dong quai - Uses, side effects, and more. (n.d.). WebMD. https://www.webmd.com/vitamins/ai/ingredientmono-936/dong-quai

Durward, E. (2022, June 20). *Is the Mediterranean diet good for menopause?* A. Vogel. https://www.avogel.co.uk/health/menopause/videos/is-the-mediterranean-diet-good-for-menopause/

Dweck, A. (2022, June 20). The Mediterranean diet & eating well for menopause. *Bonafide*. https://hellobonafide.com/blogs/news/the-mediterranean-diet-and-dietary-supplements-for-menopause

Ehsanpour, S., Salehi, K., Zolfaghari, B., & Bakhtiari, S. (2012). The effects of red clover on quality of life in post-menopausal women. *Iranian journal of nursing and midwifery research, 17*(1), 34–40. https://www.ncbi.nlm.nih.gov/pmc/articles/PMC3590693/

8 ingredients to glowing skin during menopause. (2022, October 12). Advanced Nutrition Programme. https://advancednutritionprogramme.com/nutrition-edit/8-ingredients-to-glowing-skin-during-menopause-/

EliteCare Health Centers. (2023, August 30). 7 ways to manage hormonal imbalance after menopause. *EliteCare Health Centers*. https://www.elitecarehc.com/blog/7-ways-to-manage-hormonal-imbalance-after-menopause/

Elkins, G. R., Fisher, W. I., Johnson, A. K., Carpenter, J. S., & Keith, T. Z. (2013). Clinical hypnosis in the treatment of postmenopausal hot flashes. Menopause: *The journal of the North American Menopause Society, 20*(3), 291–298. https://doi.org/10.1097/gme.0b013e31826ce3ed

Feduniw, S., Korczyńska, L., Górski, K., Zgliczyńska, M., Bączkowska, M., Byrczak, M., Kociuba, J., Ali, M., & Ciebiera, M. (2022). The effect of vitamin E supplementation in postmenopausal women—A systematic review. *Nutrients, 15*(1), 160. https://doi.org/10.3390/nu15010160

Felipe, J., Viezel, J., Dias Reis, A., da Costa Barros, E. A., de Paulo, T. R. S., Neves, L. M., & Freitas, I. F., Jr. (2020). Relationship of different intensities of physical activity and quality of life in postmenopausal women. *Health and quality of life outcomes, 18*(1). https://doi.org/10.1186/s12955-020-01377-1

Female peptide therapy. (n.d.). Starsiak Aesthetics. https://www.starsiakaesthetics.com/treatments/female-peptide-therapy/

Flaxseed oil benefits & side effects. (2019, March 28). Ayur Times. https://www.ayurtimes.com/flaxseed-oil-benefits-side-effects/

Flaxseed - Uses, side effects, and more. (n.d.). WebMD. https://www.webmd.com/vitamins/ai/ingredientmono-991/flaxseed

Forman, T. (2017, December 13). *Self-care is not an indulgence. It's a discipline*. Forbes. https://www.forbes.com/sites/tamiforman/2017/12/13/self-care-is-not-an-indulgence-its-a-discipline/?sh=28a4dcf0fee0

Freeman, E. W., Sammel, M. D., & Sanders, R. J. (2014). Risk of long-term hot flashes after natural menopause: Evidence from the Penn Ovarian Aging Study cohort. *Menopause, 21*(9), 924–932. https://doi.org/10.1097/GME.0000000000000196

Gallagher, G. (2022, July 18). *Understanding how your skin changes during menopause*. Healthline. https://www.healthline.com/health/beauty-skin-care/menopause-skin-changes

Giosuè, A., Calabrese, I., Vitale, M., Riccardi, G., & Vaccaro, O. (2022). Consumption of dairy foods and cardiovascular disease: A systematic review. *Nutrients, 14*(4), 831. https://doi.org/10.3390/nu14040831

Goulding, P. (2022, September 2). *What is interval training?* Nuffield Health. https://www.nuffieldhealth.com/article/what-is-interval-training

Gotter, A. (2023, February 16). *Essential oils for hair*. Healthline. https://www.healthline.com/health/essential-oils-for-hair-growth

Grimley, A. (n.d.). *Homeopathy for menopause, Siobhan Daffy LBSH ISHom Dip Kin.* My Second Spring. https://mysecondspring.ie/menopause-treatments-and-therapies/homeopathy-andmenopause

Groves, M. (2023, December 4). *Menopause diet: How what you eat affects your symptoms.* Healthline. https://www.healthline.com/nutrition/menopause-diet

Gunnars, K. (2023, May 3). *22 high fiber foods you should eat.* Healthline. https://www.healthline.com/nutrition/22-high-fiber-foods

Harvard Health Publishing. (2014, March 9). *Vitamin A and your bones.* https://www.health.harvard.edu/newsletter_article/vitamin-a-and-your-bones

Harvard Health Publishing. (2020a, February 1). *What's the beef with red meat?* https://www.health.harvard.edu/staying-healthy/whats-the-beef-with-red-meat

Harvard Health Publishing. (2020b, March 1). *Menopause and mental health.* https://www.health.harvard.edu/womens-health/menopause-and-mental-health

Harvard Health Publishing. (2021, February 15). *Why stress causes people to overeat.* https://www.health.harvard.edu/staying-healthy/why-stress-causes-people-to-overeat

Harvard Health Publishing. (2022, February 2). *How much calcium do you really need?* https://www.health.harvard.edu/staying-healthy/how-much-calcium-do-you-really-need#Why%20Is%201

Harvard Health Publishing. (n.d.). *A guide to women's health: Fifty and forward.* https://www.health.harvard.edu/womens-health/a-guide-to-womens-health-fifty-and-forward

Healthy eating as you age: Know your food groups. (n.d.). National Institute on Aging. https://www.nia.nih.gov/health/healthy-eating-nutrition-and-diet/healthy-eating-you-age-know-your-food-groups

Heitz, D. (2019, April 1). *Why is dong quai called the 'female ginseng'?* Healthline. https://www.healthline.com/health/dong-quai-ancient-mystery

Herndon, J. (2021, July 13). *What is sepia homeopathy?* Healthline. https://www.healthline.com/health/sepia-homeopathy

Hirata, J. D., Swiersz, L. M., Zell, B., Small, R., & Ettinger, B. (1997). Does dong quai have estrogenic effects in postmenopausal women? A double-blind, placebo-controlled trial. *Fertility and sterility, 68*(6), 981–986. https://doi.org/10.1016/s0015-0282(97)00397-x

Hogan, A. (2022, June 21). *The top ingredients to look for in menopausal skin-care.* NewBeauty. https://www.newbeauty.com/best-menopause-skin-care-ingredients/

Holland, K. (2020, August 12). *Mental health, depression, and menopause.* Healthline. https://www.healthline.com/health/menopause/mental-health

Homeostasis. (n.d.). BYJU'S. https://byjus.com/biology/homeostasis/

Hormone replacement therapy (HRT). (2022, May). Royal Osteoporosis Society. https://theros.org.uk/information-and-support/osteoporosis/treatment/hormone-replacement-therapy/

Hot flashes: What can I do? (n.d.). National Institute on Aging. https://www.nia.nih.gov/health/menopause/hot-flashes-what-can-i-do

How menopause affects your mental health. (n.d.). *Association for Women's Health Care.* https://www.chicagoobgyn.com/blog/how-menopause-affects-your-mental-health

How to combat menopausal brain fog. (2022, October 17). *Healthdirect.* https://www.healthdirect.gov.au/blog/how-to-combat-menopausal-brain-fog

Hunter, M. (n.d.). Cognitive behaviour therapy for hot flashes. *Health & Her.* https://healthandher.com/en-us/blogs/expert-advice/cognitive-behaviour-therapy-for-hot-flushes

Hunter, M. S., & Chilcot, J. (2021). Is cognitive behaviour therapy an effective option for women who have troublesome menopausal symptoms? *British journal of health psychology, 26*(3), 697–708. https://doi.org/10.1111/bjhp.12543

Hurwitz, J. M., & Santoro, N. (2004). Inhibins, activins, and follistatin in the aging female and male. *Seminars in reproductive medicine, 22*(3), 209–217. https://doi.org/10.1055/s-2004-831896

Institute of Medicine. (2001). *Dietary reference intakes: Proposed definition of dietary fiber.* National Academies Press (US). https://nap.nationalacademies.org/read/10161/chapter/1

Institute of Medicine. (2010). *Strategies to reduce sodium intake in the United States.* The National Academies Press. https://doi.org/10.17226/12818

Jack, C. (2020, May 24). Can hypnotherapy help me during menopause? *Psychology Today.* https://www.psychologytoday.com/us/blog/women-autism-spectrum-disorder/202005/can-hypnotherapy-help-me-during-menopause

Johnson, A., Roberts, L., & Elkins, G. (2019). Complementary and alternative medicine for menopause. *Journal of evidence-based integrative medicine, 24.* https://doi.org/10.1177/2515690X19829380

Jones, B. (2023, October 17). *Ways to relax during menopause.* Verywell Health. https://www.verywellhealth.com/menopause-relaxation-techniques-5219886

Kazemi, F., Masoumi, S. Z., Shayan, A., & Oshvandi, K. (2021). The effect of evening primrose oil capsule on hot flashes and night sweats in post-menopausal women: A single-blind randomized controlled trial. *Journal of menopausal medicine, 27*(1), 8–14. https://doi.org/10.6118/jmm.20033

Khadivzadeh, T., Najafi, M. N., Ghazanfarpour, M., Irani, M., Dizavandi, F. R., & Shariati, K. (2018). Aromatherapy for sexual problems in menopausal women: A systematic review and meta-analysis. *Journal of menopausal medicine, 24*(1), 56–61. https://doi.org/10.6118/jmm.2018.24.1.56

Kim, M.-J., Cho, J., Ahn, Y., Yim, G., & Park, H.-Y. (2014). Association between physical activity and menopausal symptoms in perimenopausal women. *BMC women's health*, *14*(1). https://doi.org/10.1186/1472-6874-14-122

Kimberg, T. (2023, June 30). *The silent struggle: Unveiling the effects of menopause on relationships*. LinkedIn. https://www.linkedin.com/pulse/silent-struggle-unveiling-effects-menopause-tracy-kimberg-

Know your remedy: Lachesis. (n.d.). Homeopathy Plus. https://homeopathyplus.com/know-your-remedies-lachesis-muta-lach/#General%20Information

Kołodyńska, G., Zalewski, M., & Rożek-Piechura, K. (2019). Urinary incontinence in postmenopausal women — causes, symptoms, treatment. *Menopause review*, *18*(1), 46–50. https://doi.org/10.5114/pm.2019.84157

Kubala, J. (2023a, April 24). *Vitamin A: Benefits, deficiency, toxicity, and more*. Healthline. https://www.healthline.com/nutrition/vitamin-a

Kubala, J. (2023b, May 2). *Whole-foods, plant-based diet: A detailed beginner's guide*. Healthline. https://www.healthline.com/nutrition/plant-based-diet-guide

Lambert, D. (2021, November 15). *Can herbs and spices lower blood pressure?* Medical News Today. https://www.medicalnewstoday.com/articles/can-herbs-and-spices-lower-blood-pressure

Leech, J. (2023, February 3). *11 proven benefits of olive oil*. Healthline. https://www.healthline.com/nutrition/11-proven-benefits-of-olive-oil

Let's get to the facts: Does vitamin E really help with hot flashes? (n.d.). *Kindra*. https://ourkindra.com/blogs/journal/lets-get-to-the-facts-does-vitamin-e-really-help-with-hot-flashes

Limit red and processed meat. (n.d.). World Cancer Research Fund International. https://www.wcrf.org/diet-activity-and-cancer/cancer-prevention-recommendations/limit-red-and-processed-meat/

Lordan, R., Tsoupras, A., Mitra, B., & Zabetakis, I. (2018). Dairy fats and cardiovascular disease: Do we really need to be concerned? *Foods*, *7*(3), 29. https://doi.org/10.3390/foods7030029

Lynch, L. (2022, September 26). How to support someone going through menopause. *Medichecks*. https://www.medichecks.com/blogs/menopause/how-to-support-someone-going-through-menopause

The 'M' word: supporting menopausal people in the workplace. (n.d.). *TestGorilla*. https://www.testgorilla.com/blog/supporting-menopausal-people-workplace/

Maintaining a healthy weight. (n.d.). National Institute on Aging. https://www.nia.nih.gov/health/healthy-eating-nutrition-and-diet/maintaining-healthy-weight

Mayer, B. A. (2022, September 1). *Dermatologists share skin care tips for menopause and beyond*. Healthline. https://www.healthline.com/health/beauty-skin-care/dermatologists-share-skin-care-tips-for-menopause-and-beyond

Mayo Clinic Staff. (2022a February 11). *Oophorectomy (ovary removal surgery)*. Mayo

Clinic. https://www.mayoclinic.org/tests-procedures/oophorectomy/about/pac-20385030

Mayo Clinic Staff. (2022b December 9). *Meatless meals: The benefits of eating less meat.* Mayo Clinic. https://www.mayoclinic.org/healthy-lifestyle/nutrition-and-healthy-eating/in-depth/meatless-meals/art-20048193

Mayo Clinic Staff. (2023a, May 25). *Menopause - Diagnosis and treatment.* Mayo Clinic. https://www.mayoclinic.org/diseases-conditions/menopause/diagnosis-treatment/drc-20353401

Mayo Clinic Staff (2023b, May 25). *Menopause - Symptoms and causes.* Mayo Clinic. https://www.mayoclinic.org/diseases-conditions/menopause/symptoms-causes/syc-20353397

Mayo Clinic Staff. (2023c, May 25). *Perimenopause - Symptoms and causes.* Mayo Clinic. https://www.mayoclinic.org/diseases-conditions/perimenopause/symptoms-causes/syc-20354666

Mayo Clinic Staff. (2023d, August 10). *Vitamin E.* Mayo Clinic. https://www.mayoclinic.org/drugs-supplements-vitamin-e/art-20364144

Mayo Clinic Staff. (2023e, December 12). *Hot flashes - Symptoms and causes.* Mayo Clinic. https://www.mayoclinic.org/diseases-conditions/hot-flashes/symptoms-causes/syc-20352790

McDermott, A. (2023, June 26). *Can vitamins help alleviate my menopause symptoms?* Healthline. https://www.healthline.com/health/menopause/vitamins-for-menopause

Menopausal symptoms: In depth. (2017, May). National Center for Complementary and Integrative Health (NCCIH). https://www.nccih.nih.gov/health/menopausal-symptoms-in-depth

Menopause. (2022, January 24). Endocrine Society. https://www.endocrine.org/patient-engagement/endocrine-library/menopause

Menopause. (n.d.). Mount Sinai Health System. https://www.mountsinai.org/health-library/report/menopause

Menopause and osteoporosis. (n.d.). Better Health Channel. https://www.betterhealth.vic.gov.au/health/conditionsandtreatments/menopause-and-osteoporosis

Menopause and weight. (n.d.). Better Health Channel. https://www.betterhealth.vic.gov.au/health/conditionsandtreatments/menopause-and-weight-gain

Menopause and your heart. (n.d.). British Heart Foundation. https://www.bhf.org.uk/informationsupport/support/women-with-a-heart-condition/menopause-and-heart-disease

Menopause and your mental wellbeing. (2022, November 29.). NHS Inform. https://www.nhsinform.scot/healthy-living/womens-health/later-years-around-50-

years-and-over/menopause-and-post-menopause-health/menopause-and-
your-mental-wellbeing/

Menopause decoded. (n.d.). My Menopause Centre. https://www.mymenopausecen
tre.com/video/menopause-decoded/

Menopause incontinence. (n.d.). Stella. https://www.onstella.com/menopause-symp
toms/menopause-and-urinary-incontinence/

Merz, B. (2017, March 20). *Nonhormonal treatments for menopause.* Harvard Health
Publishing. https://www.health.harvard.edu/womens-health/nonhormonal-
treatments-for-menopause

Mind-body connection: What is it and how to strengthen it. (2023, November 13).
Calm Team Blog. https://www.calm.com/blog/mind-body-connection

Mind Tools Content Team. (n.d.). *Achieving personal empowerment.* Mind Tools.
https://www.mindtools.com/aiaydss/achieving-personal-empowerment

Mishra, N., Mishra, V. N., & Devanshi. (2011). Exercise beyond menopause: Dos
and don'ts. *Journal of mid-life health, 2*(2), 51-56. https://doi.org/10.4103/0976-
7800.92524

Mohapatra, S., Iqubal, A., Ansari, M. J., Jan, B., Zahiruddin, S., Mirza, M. A.,
Ahmad, S., & Iqbal, Z. (2022). Benefits of black cohosh (Cimicifuga racemosa)
for women health: An up-close and in-depth review. *Pharmaceuticals, 15*(3), 278.
https://doi.org/10.3390/ph15030278

Nadeem, H. (2023, February 23). What are the 34 symptoms of menopause? *Revive
Research Institute, LLC.* https://www.reviveresearch.org/blog/what-are-the-34-
symptoms-of-menopause/

Nall, R. (2023a, May 17). *Comparing premenopause and perimenopause.* Medical
News Today. https://www.medicalnewstoday.com/articles/318660#peri
menopause-and-beyond

Nall, R. (2023b, December 6). *What are the vasomotor symptoms of menopause?* Medical
News Today. https://www.medicalnewstoday.com/articles/317801#risk-factors

NAMS. (n.d.-a). *Changes in hormone levels.* The North American Menopause Society. https://www.menopause.org/for-women/sexual-health-menopause-
online/changes-at-midlife/changes-in-hormone-levels

NAMS. (n.d.-b). *Five solutions for menopause symptoms.* North American Menopause
Society. https://www.menopause.org/for-women/menopauseflashes/
menopause-symptoms-and-treatments/five-solutions-for-menopause-
symptoms

NHS. (n.d.-a). *Symptoms—Menopause.* https://www.nhs.uk/conditions/
menopause/symptoms/

NHS. (n.d.-b). *Treatment—Menopause.* https://www.nhs.uk/conditions/
menopause/treatment/

NHS. (n.d.-c). *Types of hormone replacement therapy (HRT)*. https://www.nhs.uk/medicines/hormone-replacement-therapy-hrt/types-of-hormone-replacement-therapy-hrt/

9 ways to empower yourself during the perimenopause. (n.d.). *The Marion Gluck Clinic*. https://www.mariongluckclinic.com/blog/9-ways-to-empower-yourself-during-the-perimenopause.html

The North American Menopause Society (NAMS). (2015). Nonhormonal management of menopause-associated vasomotor symptoms. *Menopause 2*,(11), 1155-1174. https://doi.org/10.1097/GME.0000000000000546

Nuts and seeds. (n.d.). Better Health Channel. https://www.betterhealth.vic.gov.au/health/healthyliving/Nuts-and-seeds

Oakley, J. (2021, November 11). Why self care is so important during menopause? *Scentered*. https://scentered.com/blogs/news/why-self-care-is-so-important-during-menopause

O'Brien, S. (2023, February 3). *Lentils: Nutrition, benefits, and how to cook them.* Healthline. https://www.healthline.com/nutrition/lentils

Otte, J. L., Carpenter, J. S., Roberts, L., & Elkins, G. R. (2020). Self-hypnosis for sleep disturbances in menopausal women. *Journal of women's health, 29*(3), 461–463. https://doi.org/10.1089/jwh.2020.8327

Payette, J. R. (n.d.). *Jennifer Ritchie Payette quotes*. Goodreads.

Payne, J. M. (2021, February 18). *Why you should exercise your way through menopause*. Penn Medicine Lancaster General Health. https://www.lancastergeneralhealth.org/health-hub-home/2021/february/why-you-should-exercise-your-way-through-menopause

Petrullo, L. (2023, February 9). An A to Z guide on antioxidants for skin. *Asian Beauty Essentials*. https://asianbeautyessentials.com/blogs/the-idol-beauty-blog/antioxidants-for-skin

Physiopedia Contributors. (n.d.). *Menopause associated arthralgia*. Physiopedia. https://www.physio-pedia.com/index.php?title=Menopause_Associated_Arthralgia&oldid=341494

Piccolo, P. (2023, June). The unspoken whispers: Perimenopause/menopause in the workplace and the tale of "We don't talk about Bruno." *Piccolo Heath LLP*. https://www.piccoloheath.com/blog/the-unspoken-whispers-perimenopause/menopause-in-the-workplace-and-the-tale-of-we-dont-talk-about-bruno

Pugle, M. (2021, June 29). *Symptoms of premenopause*. Verywell Health. https://www.verywellhealth.com/premenopausal-symptoms-5185214

Red clover. (n.d.-a). Mount Sinai Health System. https://www.mountsinai.org/health-library/herb/red-clover

Red clover. (n.d.-b). RxList. https://www.rxlist.com/red_clover/generic-drug.htm

Red clover - Uses, side effects, and more. (n.d.). WebMD. https://www.webmd.com/vitamins/ai/ingredientmono-308/red-clover

Roach, H. (n.d.). *Mediterranean diet for menopause.* Health & Her. https://healthand her.com/expert-advice/weight-gain/mediterranean-diet-menopause/

Rodolfo, K. (2000, January 3). *What is homeostasis?* Scientific American. https://www.scientificamerican.com/article/what-is-homeostasis/

Rose, H. (2023, April 28). Self-care for menopause: How can I help myself during menopause? *Calmerry Blog.* https://calmerry.com/blog/self-care/self-care-for-menopause-how-can-i-help-myself-during-menopause/

Ryczkowska, K., Adach, W., Janikowski, K., Banach, M., & Bielecka-Dabrowa, A. (2023). Menopause and women's cardiovascular health: is it really an obvious relationship? *Archives of medical science: AMS, 19*(2), 458–466. https://doi.org/10.5114/aoms/157308

Saljoughian, M. (2018, January 19). *Menopause: Changes and challenges.* U.S. Pharmacist. https://www.uspharmacist.com/article/menopause-changes-and-challenges

Santen, R. J., & Loprinzi, C. S. (2023, October 24). *Patient education: Non-estrogen treatments for menopausal symptoms (beyond the basics).* UpToDate. https://www.uptodate.com/contents/non-estrogen-treatments-for-menopausal-symptoms-beyond-the-basics/print

Sathyapalan, T., Aye, M., Rigby, A. S., Thatcher, N. J., Dargham, S. R., Kilpatrick, E. S., & Atkin, S. L. (2018). Soy isoflavones improve cardiovascular disease risk markers in women during the early menopause. *Nutrition, metabolism & cardiovascular diseases, 28*(7), 691–697. https://doi.org/10.1016/j.numecd.2018.03.007

Scott, E. (2021, September 13). *Body scan meditation.* Verywell Mind. https://www.verywellmind.com/body-scan-meditation-why-and-how-3144782

Self-care in perimenopause — and why it's so important in our 40s during. (n.d.). Women Living Better. https://womenlivingbetter.org/self-care/

Sharma, V. (n.d.-a). *Beat your climacteric blues with natural homeopathic remedies for menopause.* Dr. Homeo. https://www.drhomeo.com/menopause/homeopathic-remedies-for-menopause/

Sharma, V. (n.d.-b). *Phosphorus — Homeopathic medicine: Its uses, indications and dosage.* Dr. Homeo. https://www.drhomeo.com/medicine/phosphorus-homeo pathic-medicine/

Shoemaker, S. (2024, January 11). *Your guide to black cohosh.* Healthline. https://www.healthline.com/health/food-nutrition/black-cohosh

Shotter, S. (2022, October 24). *If you're going through menopause, these are the skincare ingredients you should be using.* Dr. Sophie Shotter. https://drsophieshotter.

com/if-youre-going-through-menopause-these-are-the-skincare-ingredients-you-should-be-using/

Shuckburgh, L. (2023, August 29). *Elevating success, the importance of menopause awareness at work.* LinkedIn. https://www.linkedin.com/pulse/elevating-success-importance-menopause-awareness-work-shuckburgh/

Siegmund-Roach, S. (2015, April 6). A guide to essential oil safety. *The Herbal Academy Blog.* https://theherbalacademy.com/a-guide-to-essential-oil-safety/

Silva-Santos, T., Moreira, P., Rodrigues, M., Padrão, P., Pinho, O., Norton, P., Ndrio, A., & Gonçalves, C. (2022). Interventions that successfully reduced adults salt intake—A systematic review. *Nutrients, 14*(1), 6. https://doi.org/10.3390/nu14010006

Skin care during menopause. (2023, March 3). *Meder Beauty.* https://mederbeauty.com/blogs/blog/skin-care-during-menopause

Smith, L. (n.d.). *How to support someone during the menopause.* Patient. https://patient.info/news-and-features/how-to-support-someone-during-the-menopause

Sood, R., Kuhle, C. L., Kapoor, E., Thielen, J. M., Frohmader, K. S., Mara, K. C., & Faubion, S. S. (2019). Association of mindfulness and stress with menopausal symptoms in midlife women, *Climacteric, 22*(4), 377-382. https://doi.org/10.1080/13697137.2018.1551344

Sowers, M. F. R., Eyvazzadeh, A. D., McConnell, D., Yosef, M., Jannausch, M. L., Zhang, D., Harlow, S., & Randolph, J. F., Jr. (2008). Anti-mullerian hormone and inhibin B in the definition of ovarian aging and the menopause transition. *The Journal of clinical endocrinology and metabolism, 93*(9), 3478–3483. https://doi.org/10.1210/jc.2008-0567

Spritzler, F., & Kubala, J. (2024, January 17). *What are the symptoms of too much vitamin D?* Healthline. https://www.healthline.com/nutrition/vitamin-d-side-effects

Sternfeld, B., & Dugan, S. (2011). Physical activity and health during the menopausal transition. *Obstetrics and gynecology clinics of North America, 38*(3), 537–566. https://doi.org/10.1016/j.ogc.2011.05.008

Stöppler, M. C. (n.d.). *Night sweats.* MedicineNet. https://www.medicinenet.com/night_sweats/article.htm

Su, H. I., & Freeman, E. W. (2009). Hormone changes associated with the menopausal transition. *Minerva ginecol, 61*(6), 483–489. https://www.ncbi.nlm.nih.gov/pmc/articles/PMC3823936/

Sung, M.-K., Lee, U. S., Ha, N. H., Koh, E., & Yang, H.-J. (2020). A potential association of meditation with menopausal symptoms and blood chemistry in healthy women: A pilot cross-sectional study. *Medicine, 99*(36), e22048. https://doi.org/10.1097/MD.0000000000022048

Symptoms. (n.d.). Rock My Menopause. https://rockmymenopause.com/get-informed/symptoms/

Tai Chi for menopause symptoms. (n.d.). Just Breathe. https://justbreathetaichi.com/2023/02/tai-chi-for-menopause-symptoms/

Tamira Scientific Committee. (2023, September 1). How to deal with pigmentation due to hormonal imbalance? *Tamira Life.* https://www.tamiralife.com/blog/how-to-deal-with-pigmentation-due-to-hormonal-imbalance

31 high-fiber foods you should be eating. (2023, March 9). Cleveland Clinic. https://health.clevelandclinic.org/high-fiber-foods

Townley, C. (2019, January 29). *Menopause: Mindfulness may reduce symptoms.* Medical News Today. https://www.medicalnewstoday.com/articles/324279#Mindfulness-as-a-treatment

2015–2020 dietary guidelines. (n.d.). U.S. Department of Health and Human Services. https://health.gov/our-work/food-nutrition/previous-dietary-guidelines/2015

Types of hormone therapy. (n.d.). Mount Sinai Health System. https://www.mountsinai.org/health-library/special-topic/types-of-hormone-therapy

Villines, Z. (2020, March 12). *Essential oils and menopause: Can they help?* Medical News Today. www.medicalnewstoday.com/articles/317918

Vitamin B6. (n.d.). Drugs.com. https://www.drugs.com/mtm/vitamin-b6.html

Vitamin B12 deficiency. (n.d.). Cleveland Clinic. https://my.clevelandclinic.org/health/diseases/22831-vitamin-b12-deficiency

Vitamin B12 side effects. (n.d.). Drugs.com. https://www.drugs.com/sfx/vitamin-b12-side-effects.html#other-side-effects

Warwick, J. (2023, October 13). *A new chapter: Menopause and its impact on relationships.* Counselling Directory. https://www.counselling-directory.org.uk/memberarticles/a-new-chapter-menopause-and-its-impact-on-relationships

WebMD Editorial Contributors. (n.d.-a). *Health benefits of evening primrose oil.* WebMD. https://www.webmd.com/diet/health-benefits-evening-primrose-oil

WebMD Editorial Contributors. (n.d.-b). *Learning to relax during menopause.* WebMD. https://www.webmd.com/menopause/learning-relax-during-menopause

WebMD Editorial Contributors. (n.d.-c). *Menopause and good nutrition.* WebMD. https://www.webmd.com/menopause/staying-healthy-through-good-nuitrition

WebMD Editorial Contributors. (n.d.-d). *Natural treatments for menopause symptoms.* WebMD. https://www.webmd.com/menopause/menopause-natural-treatments

WebMD Editorial Contributors. (n.d.-e). *Perimenopause.* WebMD. https://www.webmd.com/menopause/guide-perimenopause

WebMD Editorial Contributors. (n.d.-f). *What are the side effects of vitamin D?* WebMD. https://www.webmd.com/vitamins-and-supplements/what-are-the-side-effects-of-vitamin-d

WebMD Editorial Contributors. (n.d.-g). *What to know about menopause fatigue.* WebMD. https://www.webmd.com/healthy-aging/what-to-know-about-menopause-fatigue

What is menopause? (n.d.). National Institute on Aging. https://www.nia.nih.gov/health/menopause/what-menopause

What is the mind-body connection? (2019, October 7). Newport Academy. https://www.newportacademy.com/resources/mental-health/understanding-the-mind-body-connection/

Whiteley, C. (n.d.). *Menopause exercise: The top 5 best exercises.* Health & Her. https://healthandher.com/us/hot-topics/best-exercises-for-menopause/

Why exercising after menopause is important—and how you should do it. (n.d.). All About Women Obstetrics and Gynecology. https://www.allaboutwomenmd.com/knowledge-center/exercise-after-menopause.html

Wilkinson, L. (n.d.). *HRT and testosterone - what you need to know.* Stella. https://www.onstella.com/the-latest/hrt/hrt-and-testosterone/

Worden, J. (n.d.). *Menopausal symptoms.* Homeopathy UK. https://homeopathy-uk.org/conditions-directory/menopausal-symptoms/

World Health Organization. (2022, October 17). *Menopause.* https://www.who.int/news-room/fact-sheets/detail/menopause

Yang, Y. J. (2019). An overview of current physical activity recommendations in primary care. *Korean journal of family medicine, 40*(3), 135–142. https://doi.org/10.4082/kjfm.19.0038

Yazdkhasti, M., Simbar, M., & Abdi, F. (2015). Empowerment and coping strategies in menopause women: A review. *Iranian Red Crescent medical journal, 17*(3). https://doi.org/10.5812/ircmj.18944

Yeager, S. (2022, May 10). Another reason to eat more carbs: Fiber. *Feisty Menopause.* https://www.feistymenopause.com/blog/another-reason-to-eat-more-carbs-fiber

Younkin, L. (2023, August 2). *The 7 best supplements for menopause, according to a dietician.* Verywell Health. https://www.verywellhealth.com/best-supplements-for-menopause-7505896#toc-best-overall-one-a-day-womens-menopause-multivitamin

Printed in Great Britain
by Amazon

59944328R00109